Copyright © 2024 Created by Thomas Buchheister

All rights reserved. No part of this book may be reproduced or used in any form without the publisher's written permission, except for brief quotations in a book review

Disclaimer

The information provided in this book is for general informational purposes only. It is not intended as, nor should it be considered, medical, legal, financial, or professional advice. The author and publisher of this book are not licensed healthcare or financial professionals, and the information shared here should not replace the guidance of qualified professionals.

Readers are encouraged to consult with their doctor, financial advisor, or other relevant experts before making any significant changes to their health, lifestyle, or financial plans based on the content of this book. The author and publisher are not responsible for any adverse effects, loss, or damage that may result from the use or application of the information contained within this book.

Every individual's needs and circumstances are unique, and readers are encouraged to use their own judgment and seek personalized advice tailored to their specific situation. The testimonials, stories, and examples provided in this book are illustrative and may not reflect typical experiences.

Chapter 1: Embracing the Aging Journey

Setting the Tone

Aging is a journey, not a destination. Yet, for many of us, crossing the threshold of 50 can feel like standing at a crossroads. Society often tells us that youth is beauty, and as the years go by, it's easy to feel like we're moving away from something rather than toward something new. But what if we flipped that narrative? What if we saw aging not as a series of losses, but as a time to rediscover ourselves, embrace new opportunities, and savor the richness of life with a newfound sense of confidence?

The idea of aging gracefully means different things to different people. For some, it's about staying active and maintaining physical health. For others, it's about cultivating a sense of inner peace and acceptance. And for many, it's a combination of both—finding a balance between caring for the body and nourishing the spirit. This book aims to guide you in exploring both aspects, offering practical advice for taking care of your physical self while encouraging a positive mindset that embraces the beauty and possibilities of aging.

It's no secret that our culture often glorifies youth, celebrating it in magazines, advertisements, and movies. But this obsession with youth can make it difficult to appreciate the richness that comes with age. The images we see often lack the lines of experience, the graying hair that symbolizes wisdom, and the eyes that have seen life's ups and downs. It's easy to internalize these messages and feel as though our worth diminishes as we grow older. This chapter aims to dismantle those myths and introduce a fresh perspective: that the later chapters of life can be the most fulfilling ones yet.

For many women, reaching midlife and beyond can bring a mix of emotions—relief from the pressures of younger years, but also a sense of uncertainty. What lies ahead? How do we navigate this uncharted territory? Here, we begin to answer those questions by shifting the focus from fear to curiosity, from loss to gain, and from anxiety about the future to gratitude for the present. Aging gracefully means choosing to see each day as a gift, an opportunity to live fully, and a chance to celebrate the unique beauty that comes with age.

Changing our perspective on aging starts with changing our self-talk. Instead of focusing on what we might be losing, we can start to see what we're gaining time to pursue passions, deeper connections with loved ones, and the freedom to be true to ourselves. It's about learning to accept each new line on our faces as a story well-lived, each grey hair as a sign of resilience, and each year as a new chapter filled with potential. Aging gracefully is about more than just managing the physical changes that come with time—it's about celebrating the experiences, wisdom, and strength that each year brings.

The Science of Aging

To understand the art of aging gracefully, it helps us to know a little bit about what happens to our bodies as we grow older. Aging is a natural process, influenced by both genetic and environmental factors. While we can't control the number of candles on our birthday cake, we can certainly influence how we feel as we add those candles each year. Understanding what's happening inside our bodies can help us adapt to these changes with more compassion for ourselves.

As we age, our skin undergoes changes that can be seen and felt. Collagen and elastin, two proteins that keep skin firm and elastic, start to break down, causing skin to lose some of its resilience. This can lead to wrinkles, sagging, and a general loss of the youthful glow that many of us remember. However, this doesn't mean that glowing skin is a thing of the past—far from it! With the right care and attention, skin can remain radiant and healthy at any age. In later chapters, we'll explore skincare routines and ingredients that support mature skin, helping you feel good in your skin, no matter what your age.

Beyond skin changes, aging affects our bones and muscles. After the age of 50, bone density tends to decrease, which is why women become more susceptible to osteoporosis. Muscle mass also declines with age, which can impact our strength and mobility. But with a combination of proper nutrition and regular exercise, it's possible to maintain strong bones and muscles well into our later years. In fact, many women find that staying active as they age helps them feel more energetic and capable than ever before. Later, we'll discuss exercise routines that are gentle on joints but effective for maintaining strength and flexibility.

The brain also changes as we age, but staying mentally active and engaged can keep the mind sharp. Activities like reading, puzzles, or even learning a new language have been shown to help maintain cognitive function. But equally important is the role of social interaction— maintaining connections with friends and loved ones has been linked to better mental health and a lower risk of cognitive decline. In this book, we'll dive into ways to stay socially active and keep the mind engaged, ensuring that our golden years are rich in both companionship and mental agility.

Research shows that a positive attitude toward aging can make a significant difference in how we experience it. According to a study published in *The Journal of Gerontology*, individuals who view aging positively are more likely to maintain better physical and mental health as they age. This mindset shift can help us focus less on what we're losing and more on what we're gaining—wisdom, self-assurance, and the freedom to redefine what a fulfilling life looks like. Positive thinking alone isn't a cure-all, but it does make the daily experience of aging feel lighter and more joyful.

Changing the Narrative: Redefining Beauty and Success

For too long, the media has painted aging as a battle—something to resist, to fight, to delay. But what if, instead of fighting the aging process, we leaned into it? What if we saw beauty in a face that has lived, in a body that has carried us through years of experience, and in a mind that has grown wiser with each passing decade? What if we decided that instead of viewing aging as something to be feared, we celebrated it as an integral part of our life's journey?

Redefining beauty means appreciating the qualities that come with age—character, depth, and the confidence that comes from truly knowing yourself. It means stepping away from the myth that beauty fades with age and stepping into the truth that beauty simply evolves. This is not about giving up on feeling good about how you look— far from it! It's about finding new ways to feel beautiful and focusing on the radiance that comes from self-acceptance. In fact, embracing the changes that come with age can bring a newfound sense of freedom to express yourself without worrying about others' expectations.

One way to redefine beauty is to look to the many women who have found new ways to express themselves through fashion, makeup, and personal style as they've grown older. They don't shy away from color, nor do they hide their age—they embrace it, letting their personalities shine through. Fashion becomes less about following trends and more about feeling good in your own skin. For some, that means bold patterns and statement jewelry. For others, it's about comfort and ease. The freedom to define your own style is one of the gifts of growing older, allowing you to express your inner self in a way that feels true to who you are now, not who you were in the past.

Success, too, changes its meaning as we age. For many of us, our younger years are spent chasing traditional markers of success—career achievements, financial milestones, raising a family. But what if success after 50 was about different things—like finding joy in the little moments, cultivating deep relationships, and nurturing our passions? Success can mean feeling good in our skin, laughing with friends, trying new hobbies, or simply savoring a quiet cup of tea in the morning sun. It's about setting goals that align with your values and embracing the freedom to pursue what truly matters to you.

It's time to move beyond the narrow definitions of beauty and success that have been handed down to us. This is the time to create new definitions that fit our lives, our priorities, and our dreams. As we journey through this book, we'll explore ways to cultivate a deep sense of self-worth that isn't tied to what we look like or what we achieve, but rather to who we are and the richness of our lived experiences.

Personal Reflections: Stories of Joy and Transformation

As we journey through life, each stage brings its own challenges and rewards. Many women find that their 50s and 60s become a time of profound transformation—a chance to rediscover who they are outside of the roles they've played for others. Take Maria, for example. After decades spent focusing on her career and raising her children, she found herself at a loss when she retired. But instead of letting herself feel adrift, she decided to take up watercolor painting, a hobby she had enjoyed in her youth but had put aside. Now, Maria spends her afternoons in her garden with her paints, finding peace in the colors and shapes she creates on the page. She says, "I may not be working in an office anymore, but I've found a new way to express myself. My paintings may not be masterpieces, but they make me feel alive."

Then there's Joanne, who, at 62, decided to join a local hiking group. "I thought I was too old to start something new," she admits. "But I found that walking in the woods with people who became friends, breathing in the fresh air, and challenging myself to climb hills I thought were impossible—that's where I found my confidence again." Joanne's story reminds us that it's never too late to rediscover our sense of adventure, to find new passions, and to embrace challenges that keep our spirits vibrant. Her experience reflects the power of nature and connection, showing how even a simple walk can bring a sense of renewal.

Carol's story is another example. After her husband passed away, she spent years feeling lonely and isolated. It wasn't until she started volunteering at a local community center that she found a renewed sense of purpose. "I thought my best years were behind me," she recalls. "But now, I see that I have so much to give and so much to learn. Helping others has brought me back to life." Her story shows the power of connection and the importance of staying engaged with the world around us. Volunteering allowed her to use her time and skills in new ways, transforming her grief into a renewed sense of belonging and joy.

Each of these stories shares a common theme: the realization that life doesn't stop at 50, 60, or even 70. It simply changes form, offering new possibilities that can be just as fulfilling as the ones we've left behind. These women, and many others like them, have found that the years after 50 can be a time of growth and self-discovery, even when life takes unexpected turns. The joy they've found in new hobbies, friendships, and contributions to their communities is a testament to the idea that there's no expiration date on living fully.

When we share our stories, we create a tapestry of experiences that remind us we are not alone in our journey. Hearing from others who have faced similar challenges or taken the leap into new ventures can inspire us to take our own steps forward. Throughout this book, we'll continue to hear from women who have redefined aging on their terms, turning each new chapter into an opportunity for joy and connection.

Why This Book Matters

If you've picked up this book, chances are you're looking for more than just advice—you're looking for inspiration.

You want to know that it's possible to age with grace and dignity, that it's possible to feel beautiful and strong, even as your body changes. You want to see role models who have walked this path before you, and you want practical tips that make the journey easier. This book aims to provide both inspiration and practical guidance, blending expert advice with personal stories that show the beauty of aging.

In the pages that follow, we'll explore ways to care for your body, nourish your mind, and embrace your spirit. From skincare routines that celebrate mature beauty to exercise tips that keep you moving with ease, this book is your companion in embracing the art of aging gracefully. The advice you'll find here isn't about turning back the clock, it's about finding ways to feel your best at every stage. It's about understanding the unique needs of a body that has carried you through decades and learning to care for it with the love and attention it deserves.

We'll hear from dermatologists who can explain how to adapt skincare routines to meet the needs of aging skin. We'll get insights from nutritionists on maintaining energy and vitality through diet, and from fitness coaches who will share exercises that strengthen and support the body without strain. These experts will offer practical, science-backed tips that you can easily incorporate into your daily life. But just as importantly, you'll hear the voices of women who have faced the challenges of aging with resilience and grace, sharing their stories of triumph, joy, and growth.

Aging gracefully is an art—an art that anyone can master with the right mindset and tools. This book is designed to help you find those tools, whether that means adjusting your skincare routine, finding a new passion, or simply shifting your perspective. Together, we'll redefine what it means to grow older, shifting the focus from what we leave behind to what lies ahead. We'll explore the potential for new friendships, new hobbies, and a renewed sense of purpose that can make the years ahead some of the best yet.

For too long, society has emphasized what we lose as we age: youth, flexibility, the roles that defined us for so long. But aging gracefully is about discovering what we gain. It's about finding a deeper connection to ourselves, appreciating the journey we've been on, and looking forward to the adventures still to come. It's about knowing that while we can't control every change that comes with age, we can choose how we respond to it—with grace, with humor, and with the knowledge that each year adds another layer of richness to our lives.

This book is not about striving for perfection or fitting into a mold of what aging "should" look like. It's about embracing what makes you uniquely you, at every age and every stage. It's about allowing yourself to enjoy the process, even when it means accepting changes that aren't always easy. It's about recognizing that aging is a privilege—a chance to continue growing, learning, and experiencing the world in new ways.

As you turn the pages of this book, I hope you'll feel a sense of companionship and encouragement. I hope the stories and insights here will remind you that you are not alone on this journey, and that there is a community of women who, like you, are embracing each day with openness and curiosity. Let's embark on this journey together, celebrating every wrinkle, every laugh line, and every step forward with a smile. After all, the art of aging gracefully is about seeing the beauty in every stage of life and learning to appreciate the person we are becoming.

Chapter 2: Skincare and Beauty: Nurturing the Skin You're In

Understanding Your Skin

Our skin is our largest organ, and it tells the story of our life—every smile, every moment spent in the sun, and even the stresses we've weathered along the way. As we age, our skin naturally changes, becoming thinner and less elastic. Collagen, the protein that keeps our skin firm, starts to break down, while elastin fibers, which give our skin its bounce, become less resilient. This is why we may notice fine lines, wrinkles, and a loss of firmness in our faces. But understanding these changes can help us make choices that keep our skin looking and feeling its best.

As estrogen levels decrease during menopause, our skin can become drier and more sensitive. The sebaceous glands, which produce natural oils, slow down, which can lead to a feeling of tightness and increased dryness. This shift means that the moisturizers and products that worked in our 30s and 40s may no longer be effective. Instead, it's time to focus on richer, more hydrating formulas that help restore moisture and strengthen the skin barrier. We'll dive into product recommendations later, but for now, remember hydration is your new best friend.

Sun exposure is one of the leading causes of visible aging, contributing to everything from age spots to a rougher texture. Even if you were a sun-worshiper in your youth, it's never too late to start protecting your skin. Dermatologists recommend using a broad-spectrum SPF of at least 30 every day, rain or shine. Sunscreen not only helps prevent further sun damage, but it can also reduce the risk of skin cancer, which becomes more of a concern as we age.

Another factor that influences the aging process is lifestyle. A diet high in processed foods and sugar can contribute to inflammation, which in turn can accelerate skin aging. Conversely, a diet rich in antioxidants—found in fruits, vegetables, and certain teas—can help fight free radicals, molecules that damage skin cells. The environment also plays a role, with pollution and toxins contributing to oxidative stress. That's why many dermatologists now recommend using antioxidant serums, like those containing vitamin C, as part of a daily skincare routine.

As we continue through this chapter, we'll explore how to adjust your skincare routine to meet these changes, focusing on products and habits that support your skin's health and vitality. From serums to moisturizers, and even a few natural remedies, you'll learn how to adapt your routine to ensure your skin remains a beautiful reflection of your life's journey.

Advice from Dermatologists

When it comes to understanding how to care for mature skin, dermatologists offer a wealth of knowledge that can make a significant difference in your routine. One of the most common recommendations is to prioritize hydration, especially for skin that tends to become drier with age. Dr. Jane Mitchell, a board-certified dermatologist, suggests using products that contain hyaluronic acid—a powerful ingredient that attracts moisture to the skin, keeping it plump and supple. "Hyaluronic acid is like a drink of water for your skin," she explains. "It helps to smooth out fine lines and gives your skin a hydrated, youthful appearance."

Another key recommendation is the use of retinoids, which are derived from vitamin A and known for their anti-aging benefits. Retinoids can help increase cell turnover, reduce the appearance of fine lines, and improve skin texture. Dr. Samantha Lee notes, "Retinoids are the gold standard for aging skin, but it's important to start slowly, especially if you have sensitive skin." She advises beginning with a low-strength product a few nights a week, gradually increasing frequency as your skin adjusts.

Antioxidants are also a crucial part of any skincare routine aimed at combatting the effects of aging. Vitamin C serums are particularly popular, as they help to brighten skin, fade dark spots, and protect against environmental damage. Dr. Lee recommends applying a vitamin C serum in the morning, followed by sunscreen, for optimal protection throughout the day. "Think of it as a one-two punch against free radicals," she says.

Beyond topical treatments, dermatologists often emphasize the importance of lifestyle factors. Dr. Mitchell points out that "no amount of cream can replace the benefits of healthy lifestyles like drinking plenty of water, eating a balanced diet, and getting enough sleep can have a tremendous impact on how your skin looks and feels." Staying hydrated helps maintain skin elasticity, while a diet rich in fruits, vegetables, and omega-3 fatty acids can nourish the skin from the inside out.

For those looking to address specific concerns like age spots or skin laxity, consulting with a dermatologist for personalized treatments, such as chemical peels, laser therapy, or microneedling, can be a worthwhile investment.

These treatments can provide targeted results, helping to rejuvenate the skin and give it a fresher appearance. As we explore the next sections, we'll dive into building a daily skincare routine that incorporates these expert tips.

Building a Daily Skincare Routine

A good skincare routine is like a daily ritual—one that not only keeps your skin looking its best but also allows you to take a moment for yourself. As skin changes with age, it's essential to adapt your routine to meet new needs. A daily skincare routine for mature skin should focus on three main goals: hydration, protection, and gentle renewal. Here's a step-by-step guide to building a routine that covers these bases.

Morning Routine

Start your day with a gentle cleanser that doesn't strip the skin of its natural oils. Many dermatologists recommend using a cream or hydrating gel cleanser that cleans without causing dryness. After cleansing, apply a vitamin C serum. This antioxidant helps protect the skin from environmental damage and brightens the complexion, giving skin a natural glow.

Next, layer on a moisturizer that suits your skin's needs. For mature skin, a moisturizer with hyaluronic acid or ceramides is ideal, as these ingredients help lock in moisture and repair the skin's barrier. If you have dry skin, look for a richer formula, while those with combination skin may prefer a lighter, hydrating lotion.

The final step in your morning routine is sunscreen, and this one is non-negotiable. Choose a broad-spectrum sunscreen with at least SPF 30 to protect your skin from harmful UVA and UVB rays. Sun exposure is a primary cause of premature aging, so daily protection is key, even on cloudy days. Tinted sunscreens can offer an additional boost, evening out skin tone while protecting your skin.

Evening Routine
At night, your skin shifts into repair mode, making this the time to focus on rejuvenation. Begin with a gentle cleanser to remove the day's makeup, sunscreen, and impurities. Follow up with a retinoid or retinol product. These vitamin A derivatives help increase cell turnover, smooth out fine lines, and encourage collagen production. If you're new to retinoids, start with a low-strength formula and apply it every other night to avoid irritation.

After applying retinoids, use a hydrating serum with ingredients like hyaluronic acid or peptides. These help to plump up the skin and provide moisture, countering the dryness that can sometimes accompany retinoid use. Finish your routine with a rich, nourishing moisturizer or a facial oil, especially if your skin is feeling dry or tight. Look for products containing ingredients like shea butter or squalane, which help to seal in hydration.

Weekly Treatments
In addition to your daily routine, weekly treatments can give your skin an extra boost. Exfoliating once or twice a week with a gentle chemical exfoliant, like a glycolic acid or lactic acid serum, helps to remove dead skin cells and improve skin texture. This encourages a smoother, brighter complexion without the harshness of physical scrubs that can be too abrasive for mature skin.

Masks are another great addition to a weekly routine, providing concentrated benefits. For dry skin, try a hydrating mask with ingredients like aloe vera or hyaluronic acid. For those who struggle with uneven skin tone or sunspots, a brightening mask with ingredients like vitamin C or niacinamide can be effective. Consider using a mask as a Sunday evening treat—a way to wind down and prepare your skin for the week ahead.

Consistency is Key
One of the most important aspects of a successful skincare routine is consistency. It's easy to get swept up in the latest trends or products, but sticking to a simple, targeted routine is often the most effective approach. It allows your skin to adjust to new products and minimizes the risk of irritation. Remember, it can take several weeks to start seeing results from new products, so patience is just as important as persistence.

Taking the time each morning and evening to care for your skin can be a form of self-care, a way to show yourself love and attention. A good skincare routine doesn't just improve your skin—it's a small act of kindness you can give yourself each day.

Natural Skincare Options

Natural skincare has become increasingly popular, and many people find comfort in knowing they're using ingredients derived directly from nature. For mature skin, certain natural oils and botanical extracts can offer gentle, effective benefits without the harsh chemicals that can sometimes irritate sensitive skin. Incorporating these natural options into your skincare routine can be a wonderful way to treat your skin kindly while enjoying the rich nutrients that nature provides.

Nourishing Oils for Mature Skin
Natural oils can provide deep hydration and nourishment, especially for skin that's become drier with age. Argan oil, often referred to as "liquid gold," is rich in vitamin E and essential fatty acids, making it a great option for moisturizing and softening the skin. It's lightweight enough to use during the day but hydrating enough to act as a night treatment, leaving skin feeling supple and smooth.

Rosehip oil is another favorite for aging skin, thanks to its high concentration of vitamin A and antioxidants. It's known for its ability to reduce the appearance of fine lines and scars, making it an excellent choice for those looking to smooth out their complexion. Apply a few drops of rosehip oil after your moisturizer, letting it seal in the hydration and provide an extra layer of nourishment.

For those looking to boost skin elasticity, pomegranate seed oil is a hidden gem. Rich in omega-5 fatty acids, this oil helps to rejuvenate the skin and improve its overall tone. Its anti-inflammatory properties make it ideal for sensitive skin that needs a little extra care, helping to soothe redness and irritation while supporting the skin's natural barrier.

Herbal Extracts and DIY Treatments
Herbs like chamomile, aloe vera, and green tea have long been used in skincare for their soothing properties. Aloe vera gel, for instance, is a powerful natural hydrator that helps calm irritated skin and reduce redness. It's perfect for use after sun exposure or whenever your skin feels sensitive or inflamed. Simply apply a thin layer directly from the plant or use a store-bought gel that's free from added fragrances and colors.

Green tea extract is another potent ingredient for aging skin, known for its high levels of polyphenols—compounds that have antioxidant and anti-inflammatory properties. Green tea can help protect the skin from environmental stressors while reducing puffiness and evening out skin tone. Some people enjoy using a cooled green tea bag as a quick and easy eye compress to reduce under-eye bags and refresh tired eyes.

Honey, especially raw or Manuka honey, is a natural humectant, meaning it draws moisture into the skin. Its antibacterial properties make it a gentle cleanser for those with acne-prone skin, while its soothing qualities can provide relief for dry patches. A simple DIY honey mask—apply a thin layer of honey to clean skin, leave it on for 10-15 minutes, and rinse with warm water—can leave your skin feeling soft and revitalized.

Natural Ingredients to Approach with Caution
While many natural ingredients can be beneficial, it's important to remember that "natural" doesn't always mean "gentle." Essential oils, for example, can be potent and should be used with care. Oils like tea tree, peppermint, and lavender should be diluted with a carrier oil before applying to the skin, as they can cause irritation if used undiluted.

It's also worth noting that some natural exfoliants, like sugar scrubs or crushed nut shells, can be too harsh for mature skin. These physical exfoliants can create micro-tears in the skin, leading to irritation and sensitivity. Instead, opt for gentler options like oatmeal or powdered rice, which can be mixed with honey or yogurt for a mild, homemade exfoliating mask.

Blending Nature with Science
Many skincare experts recommend combining natural products with scientifically backed ingredients like

retinoids and vitamin C. This approach allows you to enjoy the soothing and hydrating benefits of natural oils and extracts while still benefiting from the proven effects of modern skincare innovations. A routine that includes both can provide a balanced approach, helping you achieve glowing, healthy skin.

By exploring these natural options, you can create a skincare routine that feels personalized and deeply nourishing. Whether you're using a few drops of rosehip oil before bed or blending a homemade mask on the weekend, incorporating nature into your skincare routine can be a simple yet powerful way to connect with yourself and care for your skin.

Makeup Tips for Mature Skin

Makeup can be a wonderful tool for highlighting our best features, but as our skin changes with age, our approach to makeup may need a few adjustments. The key to make up for mature skin is to focus on products and techniques that enhance your natural beauty, adding a touch of radiance while avoiding heavy or cakey finishes. Here's how to adapt your makeup routine to bring out your best glow at any age.

Start with a Hydrated Base
A well-hydrated base is essential for smooth makeup application. Before applying any makeup, make sure your skin is moisturized. A hydrating primer can help create a smooth surface for foundation, filling in fine lines and giving your skin a plump, fresh appearance. Look for primers that contain ingredients like hyaluronic acid or glycerin, which attract moisture to the skin.

For those who prefer a dewy look, a lightweight facial oil can be mixed with your moisturizer or applied as a base before foundation. This adds a soft, luminous sheen that keeps the skin looking vibrant and youthful throughout the day.

Choosing the Right Foundation
When it comes to foundation, lightweight formulas are often the best choice for mature skin. A heavy, matte foundation can settle into fine lines and make skin appear dull. Instead, opt for a hydrating, medium-coverage foundation or a tinted moisturizer that evens out skin tone without masking your natural glow. Many women find that using a damp makeup sponge to apply foundation helps blend the product seamlessly, creating a natural finish.

If you prefer a little more coverage, consider using a concealer only where you need it—under the eyes, around the nose, or on any dark spots. This allows the rest of your skin to breathe while giving you a flawless look where it matters most. Choose a creamy concealer formula that won't emphasize dryness or fine lines.

Brighten Up the Eyes
As we age, the skin around the eyes can become thinner and more delicate, making dark circles and puffiness more noticeable. To brighten the eye area, use a lightweight, hydrating concealer and gently pat it in with your ring finger to avoid tugging at the skin. A touch of peach-toned corrector under the eyes can neutralize blue or purple tones, creating a more awake look.

When it comes to eyeshadow, soft, neutral shades can add definition without looking heavy. Consider using a cream shadow for a subtle wash of color that won't settle into creases. Avoid overly shimmery shadows, as these can emphasize texture on the eyelids. Instead, use a satin or matte finish that adds depth without drawing attention to fine lines.

Eyeliner can help define the eyes, but a softer approach is often more flattering. Swap harsh black liners for softer shades like brown or charcoal and try using a pencil or gel liner smudged along the lash line for a more natural look. A few coats of mascara on curled lashes can open up the eyes and create a youthful, lifted effect.

Blush and Bronzer: Adding a Natural Glow
Blush can bring a beautiful flush of color to mature skin, making it look fresh and vibrant. Cream blushes work particularly well, blending seamlessly into the skin without sitting on top of it. Choose shades that mimic a natural flush—peach, rose, or soft berry tones are universally flattering.

A touch of bronzer can also add warmth to the skin, giving it a healthy, sun-kissed look. Use a large, fluffy brush to sweep the bronzer lightly over the high points of the face, the forehead, cheeks, and jawline. This technique adds dimension without looking overdone.

Finishing Touches: Lips and Highlighter
As we age, lips can lose some of their fullness, but the right lipstick can add back definition and color. Creamy, hydrating lipsticks are a great choice, as they add moisture and comfort without settling into fine lines. Choose shades that complement your natural lip color or go for a bolder hue to make a statement.

A touch of highlighter can bring back a youthful glow to the face. Focus on applying a small amount of highlighters to the high points of the faces such as the tops of the cheekbones, the bridge of the nose, and the cupid's bow. A subtle, pearly formula can create a dewy effect without looking too shiny.

Embrace Your Individual Style
Ultimately, the best makeup is the kind that makes you feel like the best version of yourself. Whether that means a simple swipe of lipstick and mascara or a full face of glam, the most important thing is that you feel confident in your own skin. Makeup is a tool for self-expression, not a mask, and embracing your unique style is the key to aging gracefully with makeup.

Chapter 3: Nutrition: Fueling Your Body for Vitality

How Nutritional Needs Change

As we age, our bodies go through a variety of changes, and our nutritional needs shift as well. Understanding these changes can help us make better choices about what we eat, ensuring that we get the nutrients we need to stay healthy and vibrant. For women in their 50s and beyond, nutrition plays a critical role in maintaining energy, supporting bone health, and keeping our metabolism functioning optimally.

One of the most significant changes that occur with age is a slowing metabolism. This means that our bodies burn fewer calories at rest than they did in our younger years. As a result, it becomes more important to focus on nutrient-dense foods that provide a high level of vitamins and minerals without adding too many empty calories. For example, whole grains like quinoa and brown rice offer more fiber and nutrients than refined grains, making them a better choice for maintaining energy levels and digestion.

Bone health is another key concern as we get older. Women are at an increased risk for osteoporosis after menopause, due to a decrease in estrogen levels, which can lead to a loss in bone density. To support bone strength, it's crucial to get enough calcium and vitamin D. Dairy products like yogurt, milk, and cheese are well-known sources of calcium, but there are also plant-based options like almonds, chia seeds, and leafy greens such as kale and spinach. Vitamin D, often called the "sunshine vitamin," helps the body absorb calcium and can be found in foods like fatty fish, eggs, and fortified cereals, as well as supplements.

As the body ages, maintaining muscle mass becomes more challenging, but it's vital for staying active and independent. Protein plays a key role in muscle maintenance, and as we age, our bodies require more protein to repair and build muscle tissue. Incorporating high-quality protein sources into each meal—such as lean meats, fish, eggs, tofu, and legumes—can help support muscle health. Aiming for around 20-30 grams of protein per meal is a good target for most women over 50.

Digestive health can also change with age, as the digestive system slows down, making it harder to absorb certain nutrients like vitamin B12, calcium, and magnesium. This is where a diet rich in fiber can make a difference. Foods like whole grains, fruits, vegetables, and legumes are excellent sources of dietary fiber, helping to keep digestion regular and prevent constipation. Probiotic-rich foods, like yogurt, kefir, and sauerkraut, can also support gut health by maintaining a healthy balance of bacteria in the digestive system.

In addition to these physical changes, many people find that their sense of taste and appetite may change as they get older. This can be due to factors like medications or simply changes in taste buds. It's important to pay attention to these shifts and adjust meals to keep them satisfying and enjoyable. Adding herbs and spices like garlic, turmeric, and ginger can boost flavor without the need for excessive salt, which can be especially beneficial for those looking to manage blood pressure.

Hydration is another often-overlooked aspect of nutrition, but it's especially important as we age. Dehydration can occur more easily because the sensation of thirst may diminish with age, making it important to drink water regularly throughout the day, even if you don't feel thirsty. Herbal teas, infused water with fruits like lemon or berries, and eating water-rich foods like cucumbers and watermelon can help maintain hydration levels.

Understanding how these nutritional needs change the first step is toward building a diet that supports overall well-being in midlife and beyond. In the next sections, we'll look at how to put this knowledge into practice, with expert tips, meal planning ideas, and simple recipes that make healthy eating both easy and delicious.

Expert Nutrition Tips

When it comes to optimizing nutrition after 50, advice from nutrition experts can help clarify what to focus on and how to make healthy eating a sustainable habit. Here are some key insights from dietitians and nutritionists to guide you toward a balanced and nourishing diet:

1. Focus on Whole, Unprocessed Foods

Registered dietitian Sarah Nguyen emphasizes the importance of choosing whole, minimally processed foods. "As we age, our bodies benefit from foods that are as close to their natural state as possible," she says. Whole foods like fresh fruits, vegetables, whole grains, and lean proteins provide more vitamins, minerals, and fiber compared to their processed counterparts. They also tend to have less added sugar and unhealthy fats, which can contribute to inflammation in the body.

Filling half your plate with colorful fruits and vegetables is a good rule of thumb, as these foods are rich in antioxidants, which help combat oxidative stress—a key factors in the aging process. Foods like berries, leafy greens, bell peppers, and carrots are particularly high in antioxidants and can support healthy skin, immune function, and overall vitality.

2. Prioritize Protein with Each Meal

Nutritionist Dana Lopez highlights the importance of including protein in every meal. "As we age, we naturally lose muscle mass, but getting enough protein can help slow this process," she explains. Protein-rich foods like eggs, fish, poultry, beans, and legumes provide the building blocks your body needs to repair and maintain muscle. For those who prefer plant-based options, Lopez recommends incorporating tofu, tempeh, lentils, and chickpeas into meals.

A practical tip for increasing protein intake is to start the day with a protein-rich breakfast. For example, a Greek yogurt parfait with berries and nuts, or scrambled eggs with spinach and avocado, can give you a strong start to the day and keep you feeling full longer. Adding a scoop of protein powder to a smoothie is another easy way to boost your intake.

3. Embrace Healthy Fats

Many women are hesitant about fats due to outdated diet trends, but experts like Dr. Elena Martinez, a registered dietitian, emphasize that healthy fats are essential for maintaining hormonal balance and supporting brain health. "The key is to focus on sources of unsaturated fats like avocados, nuts, seeds, and olive oil," she advises. Omega-3 fatty acids, found in fatty fish, like salmon, mackerel, and sardines, are especially important as they have anti-inflammatory properties that can support heart health and joint mobility.

For those who don't eat fish regularly, Martinez suggests adding a fish oil supplement or consuming chia seeds and flaxseeds, which are plant-based sources of omega-3s. Including a small portion of healthy fats in each meal can also help you absorb fat-soluble vitamins like A, D, E, and K, which are crucial for bone health and immune function.

4. Watch Your Sugar Intake

While treats are an enjoyable part of life, it's important to be mindful of added sugars as we get older. Excessive sugar intake has been linked to increased risk of conditions like type 2 diabetes, heart disease, and weight gain. Registered dietitian Kevin Johnson suggests, "Look for ways to reduce sugar gradually—like swapping sugary drinks for sparkling water with a splash of lemon or choosing fruit for dessert instead of baked goods."

Reading food labels can be an eye-opener, as many packaged foods contain hidden sugars. Even seemingly healthy items like flavored yogurt or granola can have high sugar content. Opting for unsweetened versions and adding your own natural sweeteners, like fresh fruit or a drizzle of honey, can make a big difference.

5. Don't Forget About Hydration

Hydration becomes increasingly important as we age, yet many people find themselves drinking less water without realizing it. "Water helps keep your cells functioning properly, supports digestion, and aids in the delivery of nutrients throughout your body," says dietitian Angela Singh. She recommends aiming for at least eight 8-ounce glasses of water per day, but notes that individual needs can vary based on activity level and climate.

Singh suggests keeping a water bottle with you throughout the day as a reminder to drink. Herbal teas, like chamomile or peppermint, can be a soothing way to increase fluid intake, especially in the evening. Adding slices of lemon, cucumber, or fresh mint can make plain water more appealing.

Putting It All Together
These expert tips provide a practical framework for building a balanced diet that supports health and well-being after 50. By focusing on whole foods, prioritizing protein, including healthy fats, being mindful of sugar, and staying hydrated, you can fuel your body with what it needs to thrive. The next section will delve into how to create balanced meals, and meal plans that incorporate these principles, making it easier to enjoy nutritious food every day.

Building a Balanced Diet

Building a balanced diet is about making sure that each meal provides the nutrients your body needs to stay energized and healthy. A balanced plate is one that includes a mix of macronutrient proteins, fats, and carbohydrates— along with plenty of vitamins, minerals, and fiber. For women in their 50s and beyond, creating balanced meals can help maintain energy levels, support bone and muscle health, and promote overall well-being. Here's a guide to building a balanced diet that's easy to follow and enjoyable to maintain.

1. The Balanced Plate Approach
A simple way to structure meals is to use the "balanced

plate" method. This involves dividing your plate into three main components:

- **Half the plate filled with vegetables and fruits**: These provide essential vitamins, minerals, and antioxidants. Aim for a variety of colors, as different colors often indicate different nutrients. For example, leafy greens like spinach are rich in iron and calcium, while orange vegetables like carrots and sweet potatoes provide beta-carotene, which is important for eye health.
- **A quarter of the plate with lean protein**: Protein is crucial for maintaining muscle mass, especially as you age. This could be lean meats like chicken or turkey, fish, eggs, or plant-based sources like beans and lentils. Mixing different types of protein throughout the week keeps meals interesting and helps you get a range of nutrients.
- **A quarter of the plate with whole grains or complex carbohydrates**: Whole grains like brown rice, quinoa, and whole-wheat pasta provide long-lasting energy and help to keep blood sugar levels stable. If you're gluten-sensitive or simply want to try something different, alternatives like millet, buckwheat, or sweet potatoes can be excellent options.

2. Smart Snacking

Snacking can be a helpful way to keep your energy up between meals, but the key is to choose snacks that are both satisfying and nutritious. Opt for snacks that combine protein and healthy fats, as these can help keep hunger at bay and prevent overeating at your next meal. Good options include a handful of almonds or walnuts, apple slices with almond butter, or a piece of cheese with whole-grain crackers.

Registered dietitian Megan Simmons suggests, "Think of snacks as a way to fill in any nutritional gaps throughout the day." For example, if you didn't get enough veggies at lunch, an afternoon snack could be carrot sticks with hummus. If you're craving something sweet, try a few dark chocolate squares with fresh berries—dark chocolate is rich in antioxidants, while the berries provide a sweet, natural flavor.

3. Breakfast for a Strong Start

A balanced breakfast sets the tone for the rest of the day. Research shows that people who eat a nutritious breakfast tend to have better concentration and energy levels throughout the morning. A well-rounded breakfast includes a combination of protein, healthy fats, and complex carbohydrates. For example, overnight oats made with chia seeds, almond milk, and topped with fresh berries can provide a hearty, satisfying start to the day.

Eggs are another versatile breakfast option that's packed with protein. Pairing scrambled eggs with avocado toast or a vegetable omelet with whole-grain toast can provide a balanced meal that's easy to prepare. If you're in a rush, a smoothie with Greek yogurt, spinach, and a banana is a quick and nutrient-dense choice.

4. Dinner That Keeps You Full Without Feeling Heavy

For dinner, focusing on meals that are nourishing but not too heavy, allowing for restful sleep. A typical balanced dinner could include a piece of grilled fish, like salmon, a side of roasted vegetables, and a portion of quinoa or brown rice. Adding a leafy green salad with a simple vinaigrette provides extra fiber and helps with digestion.

Sheet pan dinners are a convenient option—try roasting chicken thighs with sweet potatoes and brussels sprouts on a single pan for an easy, one-dish meal. Adding spices like turmeric, garlic, or rosemary not only enhances flavor but also brings additional health benefits, such as reducing inflammation.

5. Planning Ahead for Success
Meal planning can make it easier to maintain a balanced diet throughout the week. Preparing meals in advance, such as batch-cooking grains, chopping vegetables, or cooking a protein to use in various meals, can save time and reduce the temptation to reach for less healthy options when you're in a rush. Having healthy staples on hand—like canned beans, frozen veggies, and whole grains—can help you put together a balanced meal even when time is tight.

Keeping a grocery list of nutrient-dense foods can help you stay on track and ensure that you have everything you need to create balanced meals. Focus on the perimeter of the grocery store, where fresh produce, lean proteins, and dairy products are typically found, while limiting visits to the aisles with highly processed foods.

Putting It All Together
Building a balanced diet doesn't have to be complicated. By focusing on whole, nutrient-rich foods and following the balanced plate method, you can ensure that each meal supports your health and well-being. The next section will provide some simple recipes that make healthy eating both delicious and easy to incorporate into your daily routine.

Recipes for Energy and Longevity

Eating well doesn't have to mean spending hours in the kitchen. Simple, nutritious recipes can be the cornerstone of a balanced diet, providing the energy you need to stay active and feel your best. Here are a few easy-to-make recipes that focus on whole ingredients, making them perfect for busy days when you still want to prioritize your health.

1. Energizing Breakfast: Blueberry Almond Overnight Oats
This easy breakfast can be made the night before, making mornings stress-free and delicious.

- **Ingredients**:
    - 1/2 cup old-fashioned oats
    - 1 tablespoon chia seeds
    - 1 cup unsweetened almond milk
    - 1/2 cup fresh or frozen blueberries
    - 1/4 teaspoon cinnamon
    - 1 tablespoon almond butter
    - 1 teaspoon honey (optional)
- **Instructions**:
    1. In a mason jar or bowl, combine oats, chia seeds, almond milk, blueberries, and cinnamon.
    2. Stir well, cover, and refrigerate overnight.
    3. In the morning, stir again and top with almond butter and a drizzle of honey if desired.
    4. Enjoy cold or heat in the microwave for a warm version.

This breakfast is packed with fiber from the oats and chia seeds, healthy fats from the almond butter, and antioxidants from the blueberries, providing long-lasting energy to start your day.

2. Light Lunch: Quinoa and Black Bean Salad
This vibrant salad is rich in protein and fiber, making it a
satisfying lunch option.

- **Ingredients**:
  - 1 cup cooked quinoa, cooled
  - 1 can (15 oz) black beans, rinsed and
    drained
  - 1 red bell pepper, diced
  - 1 cup cherry tomatoes, halved
  - 1/4 cup red onion, finely chopped
  - 1/4 cup fresh cilantro, chopped
  - Juice of 2 limes
  - 2 tablespoons olive oil
  - Salt and pepper to taste
- **Instructions**:
  1. In a large bowl, combine quinoa, black
     beans, bell pepper, cherry tomatoes, red
     onion, and cilantro.
  2. In a small bowl, whisk together lime juice,
     olive oil, salt, and pepper.
  3. Pour the dressing over the quinoa mixture
     and toss to combine.
  4. Serve chilled or at room temperature.

This salad is easy to prepare and keeps well in the fridge,
making it a great option for meal prep. The combination of
quinoa and black beans provides a complete protein source,
while the veggies add color and crunch.

3. Protein-Packed Snack: Greek Yogurt Parfait
A quick and easy snack that combines protein and
antioxidants for a boost of energy.

- **Ingredients**:
  - 1 cup plain Greek yogurt

o   1/2 cup mixed fresh berries (such as strawberries, raspberries, and blueberries)
o   1 tablespoon chopped walnuts or almonds
o   1 teaspoon honey or maple syrup (optional)

- **Instructions**:
  1. In a small bowl or glass, layer half of the Greek yogurt, followed by half of the berries.
  2. Repeat the layers with the remaining yogurt and berries.
  3. Top with chopped nuts and drizzle with honey or maple syrup if desired.

Greek yogurt is high in protein and calcium, while the berries provide antioxidants. This parfait is a great way to satisfy your sweet tooth without added sugars, making it a perfect mid-afternoon pick-me-up.

4. Nourishing Dinner: Baked Salmon with Garlic and Lemon

This simple yet flavorful dinner is rich in omega-3 fatty acids, which support heart and brain health.

- **Ingredients**:
  o   2 salmon fillets
  o   2 tablespoons of olive oil
  o   3 garlic cloves, minced
  o   Juice of 1 lemon
  o   Salt and pepper to taste
  o   Fresh parsley for garnish
- **Instructions**:
  1. Preheat the oven to 400°F (200°C).
  2. Place the salmon fillets on a lined baking sheet and drizzle with olive oil.
  3. Sprinkle with minced garlic, lemon juice, salt, and pepper.

4. Bake for 12-15 minutes, or until the salmon is opaque and flake easily with a fork.
5. Garnish with fresh parsley and serve with a side of steamed vegetables or a mixed green salad.

This baked salmon recipe is ready in under 20 minutes and pairs well with various side dishes. It's an easy way to incorporate heart-healthy fish into your diet.

5. Sweet Treat: Dark Chocolate and Nut Clusters
These simple treats offer a sweet indulgence while providing healthy fats and antioxidants.

- **Ingredients**:
    - 1 cup dark chocolate chips (70% cacao or higher)
    - 1 cup mixed nuts (almonds, walnuts, pecans)
    - Sea salt for sprinkling
- **Instructions**:
    1. Melt the dark chocolate chips in a microwave-safe bowl in 20-second intervals, stirring until smooth.
    2. Stir in the mixed nuts until evenly coated.
    3. Drop spoonsful of the mixture onto a parchment-lined baking sheet.
    4. Sprinkle with a pinch of sea salt.
    5. Refrigerate for 20 minutes or until firm.

Dark chocolate is known for its antioxidant properties, while nuts provide healthy fats and protein. These clusters make a great after-dinner treat without added sugar.

Supplements and Superfoods

While a balanced diet is the foundation of good health, there are times when supplements and superfoods can play a supportive role in maintaining vitality, especially as we age. Certain nutrients can become harder to absorb, and some superfoods offer concentrated health benefits that are worth adding to your routine. Here's a guide to some of the most beneficial supplements and superfoods for women over 50.

1. Vitamin D and Calcium

Vitamin D is essential for bone health, helping the body absorb calcium effectively. As we age, the body's ability to produce vitamin D from sunlight decreases, making supplementation an important consideration, especially for those who live in areas with limited sun exposure. A daily supplement of vitamin D3, the form that is most easily absorbed by the body, can support bone density and help prevent osteoporosis.

Calcium is equally crucial for maintaining strong bones, but getting enough from diet alone can sometimes be challenging. Dairy products, leafy greens, and fortified foods are excellent sources, but a calcium supplement can help fill any gaps. Nutritionists often recommend a combination of calcium and vitamin D supplements to ensure that both work together to support bone health.

2. Omega-3 Fatty Acids

Omega-3 fatty acids, found in fish oil and flaxseed oil, are known for their anti-inflammatory properties and their role in heart and brain health. Studies suggest that omega-3s can help reduce the risk of heart disease, improve cognitive function, and even support joint health. For those who don't consume fatty fish, like salmon, mackerel, or sardines regularly, a fish oil supplement can be a good alternative.

Vegetarians or those who prefer plant-based options can look for algae-based omega-3 supplements, which provide DHA and EPA—two types of omega-3s that are particularly beneficial. Including ground flaxseeds or chia seeds in smoothies or oatmeal can also provide a plant-based source of omega-3s, supporting heart health with every bite.

3. Probiotics for Gut Health
Gut health is closely linked to overall well-being, affecting everything from digestion to immune function. Probiotics, which are beneficial bacteria, can help maintain a healthy balance in the digestive system, especially after taking antibiotics or during times of stress. As we age, our gut microbiome can change, making probiotics a valuable addition to the diet.

Probiotic supplements often come in capsules, powders, or even as chewable tablets. Look for supplements that contain a variety of strains, such as Lactobacillus and Bifidobacterium, to ensure a broad range of benefits. Fermented foods like yogurt, kefir, sauerkraut, and kimchi are natural sources of probiotics and can be a great addition to meals, supporting digestive health in a delicious way.

4. Superfoods: Turmeric, Berries, and Greens
Certain superfoods are known for their potent health benefits and can be easily incorporated into a daily diet. Turmeric, for example, is rich in curcumin, a compound with powerful anti-inflammatory properties. Turmeric supplements can be especially beneficial for those with joint pain or arthritis. When choosing a turmeric

supplement, look for one that includes black pepper (piperine), as this enhances the absorption of curcumin.

Berries like blueberries, raspberries, and acai are high in antioxidants, which help combat oxidative stress and support brain health. Incorporating a handful of fresh or frozen berries into breakfast or enjoying them as a snack can be a simple way to boost your antioxidant intake. For those looking for a more concentrated dose, berry powders can be mixed into smoothies or yogurt.

Dark leafy greens like kale, spinach, and moringa are nutrient-dense and provide vitamins A, C, and K, as well as iron and calcium. For those who find it challenging to include enough greens in their diet, a green superfood powder can be a convenient way to add a nutritional boost to smoothies or juices.

5. B Vitamins for Energy
B vitamins, including B12, B6, and folate, are essential for energy production and maintaining nerve function. As we age, the body's ability to absorb B12 from food can decline, making supplements a good option for many people. B12 is found naturally in animal products like meat, fish, and eggs, but vegetarians and vegans, in particular, may benefit from a B12 supplement to ensure adequate levels.

B-complex supplements, which contain a blend of B vitamins, can support overall energy levels, help manage stress, and promote cognitive health. Adding a daily B-complex supplement can be particularly helpful during times of fatigue or increased stress, providing a gentle boost to help you feel your best.

Choosing the Right Supplements
Before adding any supplements to your routine, it's important to consult with a healthcare professional to ensure they're appropriate for your individual needs. Not all supplements are necessary for everyone, and a personalized approach based on your diet, lifestyle, and health conditions can help you choose the ones that will offer the most benefit.

Supplements can never replace the benefits of a balanced diet, but when used thoughtfully, they can help fill nutritional gaps and support specific health goals. By combining these with a diet rich in superfoods, you can give your body the support it needs to stay healthy and vibrant as you age.

Chapter 4: Exercise: Staying Active and Strong

The Benefits of Exercise After 50

Staying active as we age is one of the most important ways to maintain health and well-being. Regular exercise can improve mobility, boost energy levels, and support mental health, making it a key component of aging gracefully. For women over 50, exercise isn't just about maintaining a certain weight or physique—it's about building strength, flexibility, and resilience that can make everyday activities easier and more enjoyable. Here's a closer look at some of the key benefits of staying active after 50.

1. Maintaining Muscle Mass and Bone Density

As we age, we naturally lose muscle mass—a condition known as sarcopenia. This loss of muscle can affect strength, balance, and overall mobility, increasing the risk of falls and injuries. Regular strength training, such as lifting weights or using resistance bands, can help slow this process and maintain muscle mass, ensuring that you stay strong and active. Even bodyweight exercises like squats, lunges, and push-ups can be effective at preserving muscle strength.

In addition to muscle loss, women are also at risk for decreased bone density after menopause, which can lead to osteoporosis. Weight-bearing exercises, such as walking, jogging, and dancing, help stimulate bone growth, making them crucial for bone health. Strength training also plays a role in strengthening bones, as the force exerted on the bones during weightlifting helps to stimulate new bone tissue.

2. Boosting Heart Health

Cardiovascular exercise is important for keeping the heart and lungs healthy. Activities like walking, swimming, cycling, and even gardening can help to improve circulation, lower blood pressure, and reduce the risk of heart disease. Cardiovascular exercise helps to keep the heart strong, allowing it to pump blood more efficiently and deliver oxygen to the muscles and organs.

The American Heart Association recommends at least 150 minutes of moderate-intensity aerobic activity per week, which can be broken down into 30 minutes a day, five days a week. For those who prefer shorter sessions, 10-minute increments throughout the day can be just as effective. The key is consistency—regular activity is what helps maintain heart health and overall endurance.

3. Enhancing Flexibility and Balance

Flexibility naturally decreases with age, but maintaining it is essential for avoiding injuries and staying active. Stretching exercises, yoga, and Pilates are great ways to improve flexibility, keeping the muscles limber and the joints mobile. These activities can also help to alleviate stiffness, especially in areas like the lower back, hips, and shoulders, which are common sites of tension as we age.

Balance exercises are also crucial for preventing falls, which can become more of a concern as we get older. Simple exercises like standing on one leg or practicing tai chi can improve balance and coordination. Yoga poses like tree pose or chair pose are also excellent for strengthening the core muscles that support balance. Better balance can make everyday activities—like walking upstairs or carrying groceries—safer and easier.

4. Supporting Mental Well-being

Physical activity is not just good for the body; it's also a powerful tool for mental health. Exercise releases endorphins, often referred to as "feel-good" hormones, which can help reduce stress, anxiety, and symptoms of depression. For many people, the act of moving their body—whether it's through a brisk walk in nature or a gentle yoga session—provides a much-needed mental reset and a break from daily worries.

Exercise also supports cognitive function, which is crucial as we age. Research has shown that regular physical activity can help improve memory and concentration, as well as reduce the risk of cognitive decline. Activities that require coordination and focus, such as dance classes or tennis, can be especially beneficial for keeping the mind sharp. The social aspect of group exercise can also combat feelings of isolation and loneliness, adding an important social dimension to your routine.

5. Increasing Energy and Reducing Fatigue

One of the surprising benefits of regular exercise is its ability to increase overall energy levels. While it may seem counterintuitive, moving more can actually make you feel less tired in the long run. Physical activity increases circulation and helps oxygen flow more freely throughout the body, which can improve stamina and reduce feelings of fatigue.

For those who struggle with sleep, exercise can also promote better rest. Moderate aerobic activity has been shown to improve sleep quality, helping you fall asleep faster and wake up feeling more refreshed. It's best to avoid vigorous exercise too close to bedtime, as it can be energizing, but gentle stretching or yoga can be a great way to wind down in the evening.

The Takeaway
The benefits of exercise after 50 are far-reaching, touching every aspect of physical and mental health. It's not about pushing yourself to extremes, but rather finding activities that you enjoy and can stick with over time. In the next section, we'll explore different types of exercise that suit a variety of needs, helping you build a routine that supports your goals and fits your lifestyle.

Types of Exercise for Every Body

When it comes to exercise, there's no one-size-fits-all approach, especially as we age. The best exercise routine is one that meets your unique needs, keeps you motivated, and fits comfortably into your lifestyle. Here's a look at some of the most effective types of exercise for women over 50, each offering different benefits that support overall health and well-being.

1. Strength Training: Building and Maintaining Muscle
Strength training, also known as resistance training, is crucial for maintaining muscle mass as we age. It involves using weights, resistance bands, or even your own body weight to strengthen muscles. This type of exercise helps counteract the natural loss of muscle mass that occurs with aging, known as sarcopenia, and supports bone density, reducing the risk of osteoporosis.

Exercises like squats, lunges, and push-ups can be done anywhere, while using free weights or resistance bands adds variety. If you have access to a gym, machines can provide guided resistance that's particularly helpful for beginners. Aim to incorporate strength training exercises into your routine at least two to three times per week, focusing on all major muscle groups for balanced strength.

2. Cardiovascular Exercise: Keeping the Heart Strong
Cardio exercises are those that get your heart rate up, helping to improve cardiovascular health and endurance. This type of exercise is important for maintaining a healthy weight, reducing blood pressure, and increasing overall stamina. Activities like walking, swimming, cycling, and dancing are great options, and they can be adapted to different fitness levels.

Walking is one of the most accessible forms of cardio and can be done almost anywhere. For those looking to add a bit more intensity, consider alternating between brisk walking and slower-paced intervals. Swimming is a particularly good option for those with joint issues, as it provides a low-impact workout that's gentle on the knees and back while still engaging the whole body.

3. Flexibility and Balance Exercises: Enhancing Mobility
Flexibility exercises help keep muscles and joints limber, which is key for maintaining mobility and preventing injuries. Stretching, yoga, and Pilates are all excellent ways to improve flexibility, ease muscle tension, and increase range of motion. Gentle stretches at the start and end of each workout can prevent stiffness and soreness.

Yoga is particularly popular for its ability to combine flexibility and balance training. Poses like downward-facing dog, warrior, and child's pose stretch multiple muscle groups, while balance-focused poses like tree poses help strengthen stabilizer muscles. Yoga can be tailored to suit different fitness levels, with options ranging from beginner-friendly classes to more advanced flows.

Pilates focuses on core strength, which is crucial for maintaining stability and balance as we age. A strong core supports good posture and helps prevent back pain, making everyday activities like lifting groceries or gardening easier and safer. Many Pilates exercises can be done with just a mat, making it a convenient option for home workouts.

4. Low-Impact Activities: Gentle but Effective
Low-impact exercises are ideal for those who may have joint pain or are looking for a gentler way to stay active. Activities like walking, water aerobics, tai chi, and cycling provide the benefits of movement without putting too much stress on the joints. These activities are particularly well-suited for those with conditions like arthritis, as they help keep joints mobile and muscles strong without exacerbating pain.

Water aerobics, often available at community pools, is a fun and social way to exercise. The water's buoyancy supports your body, reducing stress on joints while providing gentle resistance that can improve muscle tone. Tai chi, a form of moving meditation, focuses on slow, flowing movements that enhance balance, coordination, and relaxation, making it a great option for maintaining mental clarity as well.

5. Functional Training: Moving with Purpose
Functional training involves exercises that mimic everyday movements, helping you stay strong and capable in your daily life. These exercises often engage multiple muscle groups at once and improve coordination, balance, and strength. For example, exercises like step-ups, squats, and

farmer's carries (walking while holding weights) can improve your ability to climb stairs, carry groceries, or lift objects safely.

Functional training is particularly effective for preventing injuries and maintaining independence as we age. It can be done with minimal equipment, such as dumbbells, kettlebells, or resistance bands, making it easy to incorporate into home workouts. Many fitness classes, including those focused on older adults, incorporate functional training elements to ensure participants are ready for the physical demands of daily life.

Finding What Works for You
The most important part of any exercise routine is finding activities you enjoy. Whether it's a morning walk with a friend, a weekend bike ride, or a relaxing yoga session, the best exercises are the ones that you look forward to and that fit naturally into your lifestyle. In the next section, we'll explore some sample exercise routines that can help you get started, no matter what your fitness level.

Sample Exercise Routines

Creating a balanced exercise routine doesn't have to be complicated. The key is to include a mix of strength training, cardio, flexibility, and balance exercises throughout the week. Here are some sample routines that can help you get started, whether you're new to exercise or looking to build on your current fitness level. Each routine is designed to be adaptable, allowing you to adjust based on your needs and comfort.

1. Beginner's Routine: Easing into Activity
This routine is perfect for those who are new to exercise or getting back into it after a break. It focuses on gentle movements that build a foundation of strength, flexibility, and endurance. Aim to do this routine three times per week, with a rest day in between to allow for recovery.

- **Warm-Up (5 minutes)**: Start with a gentle walk around your home or yard, or march in place to get your blood flowing.
- **Strength (10 minutes)**: Do 2 sets of 10-12 bodyweight squats, 10 wall push-ups, and 10 seated leg lifts. Rest for 30 seconds between sets.
- **Cardio (10 minutes)**: Take a brisk walk outside or use a stationary bike at a comfortable pace.
- **Stretch (5 minutes)**: Finish with gentle stretches for the hamstrings, calves, and shoulders, holding each stretch for 15-20 seconds.

This routine is a great starting point, and as your strength and endurance improve, you can gradually increase the duration of the cardio or add light weights to the strength exercises.

2. Intermediate Routine: Building Strength and Stamina
This routine is designed for those who are already active and want to increase their strength and stamina. Aim to do this routine four times per week, alternating between strength and cardio days.

- **Strength Day**:
  - **Warm-Up (5 minutes)**: March in place or do arm circles to warm up your muscles.
  - **Strength (20 minutes)**: 3 sets of 10 dumbbell rows, 10 chair squats, and 10

standing calf raises. Use light to moderate weights.
    o **Core (5 minutes)**: Do 3 sets of 10-15 seconds of planks and side planks.
    o **Stretch (5 minutes)**: Focus on stretching the back, hips, and shoulders.
- **Cardio Day**:
    o **Warm-Up (5 minutes)**: Walk or march in place.
    o **Cardio (20 minutes)**: Alternate between 2 minutes of brisk walking and 1 minute of a faster pace or light jogging.
    o **Balance (5 minutes)**: Practice standing on one leg for 10 seconds, then switch. Repeat 5 times per leg.
    o **Stretch (5 minutes)**: Finish with stretches for the legs and back.

This intermediate routine balances muscle-building exercises with cardio to improve overall fitness and endurance. As you progress, you can increase the intensity by adding more weight or extending your cardio sessions.

3. Active Aging Routine: Staying Strong and Flexible
This routine focuses on maintaining mobility and strength for everyday activities, making it ideal for those who want to stay active and independent. It's designed to be done three to four times per week.

- **Warm-Up (5 minutes)**: Gentle shoulder rolls, ankle circles, and walking in place.
- **Strength (15 minutes)**: 3 sets of 10-15 reps of resistance band exercises, including seated rows, chest presses, and seated leg presses. Resistance bands are great for adding light resistance while being gentle on the joints.

- **Cardio (15 minutes)**: Walk at a comfortable pace or use a low-impact elliptical machine. Focus on maintaining steady breathing.
- **Flexibility (10 minutes)**: Use a yoga strap or towel for seated stretches, focusing on the hamstrings and lower back. Follow with gentle twists to improve spinal mobility.

This routine emphasizes low-impact movements that support muscle tone and flexibility without putting stress on the joints. It's ideal for maintaining a strong, healthy body as you age.

Tips for Success

- **Listen to Your Body**: Pay attention to how your body feels during and after exercise. It's normal to feel a little sore after trying something new, but sharp pain is a sign to stop and rest.
- **Modify as Needed**: All exercises can be modified to suit your comfort level. For example, if floor exercises are uncomfortable, you can perform seated versions or use a chair for support.
- **Stay Consistent**: The benefits of exercise come with consistency. Find a routine that fits your lifestyle and try to stick with it. Remember, even small amounts of movement each day can make a big difference in your overall health.

These sample routines provide a framework for staying active, whether you're just starting or looking to enhance your current fitness level. In the next section, we'll explore expert tips from fitness coaches to help you make the most of your exercise routine and stay motivated on your journey.

Expert Tips from Fitness Coaches

Staying active as we age can sometimes feel challenging, but advice from experienced fitness coaches can make it easier to develop a routine that fits your needs and keeps you motivated. Here are some expert tips from fitness professionals on how to make the most of your exercise routine after 50:

1. Focus on Form, Not Just Reps

Fitness coach Lisa Harmon emphasizes that proper form is more important than the number of repetitions when it comes to strength training. "As we get older, it's crucial to protect our joints and prevent injuries, which means paying close attention to form," she says. Using proper technique ensures that the right muscles are engaged, reducing the risk of strains or pulls. If you're new to strength training, consider working with a trainer for a few sessions to learn the correct form, or use online tutorials from reputable fitness experts.

Harmon also suggests starting with lighter weights or resistance bands to get a feel for the movements before gradually increasing the load. "It's better to do 8 controlled squats with good form than 15 fast ones that put strain on your knees," she explains. Quality over quantity is key when it comes to building strength safely.

2. Prioritize Consistency Over Intensity

Coach David Alvarez believes that the secret to long-term success is consistency, not necessarily high-intensity workouts. "It's more beneficial to do moderate exercise regularly than to push yourself too hard and burn out," he advises. Consistent, moderate exercise—like a daily walk or gentle yoga session—can have cumulative benefits for heart health, flexibility, and mental well-being.

Alvarez recommends setting realistic goals and gradually increasing the duration or intensity of workouts as your fitness improves. "It's better to start with 10 minutes a day and build up to 30 than to do too much at once and risk feeling discouraged or overwhelmed," he notes. The focus should be on creating a sustainable routine that feels good, rather than following a strict regimen that might lead to frustration.

3. Warm Up and Cool Down Are Essential
Many people tend to skip warm-up and cool-down exercises, but Coach Sarah Carter stresses that these are crucial, especially as we age. "A good warm-up helps increase blood flow to the muscles and prepares your body for exercise, which can reduce the risk of injury," she explains. A proper warm-up could include dynamic stretches like arm circles, leg swings, or a light walk for 5-10 minutes.

Cooling down is just as important. "After your workout, take the time to stretch the muscles you've worked, focusing on areas that tend to get tight, like the hamstrings and back," Carter advises. Stretching after exercise helps prevent soreness and maintains flexibility, making it easier to move comfortably throughout the day.

4. Incorporate Variety to Stay Motivated
Boredom is one of the biggest obstacles to maintaining an exercise routine, according to Coach James Lee. "Switching up your workouts can keep things interesting and prevent you from hitting a plateau," he says. Variety not only keeps your mind engaged but also challenges different muscle groups, which is key for overall fitness.

Lee suggests mixing in different activities throughout the week. For example, you might do a strength training session one day, go for a swim or a bike ride the next, and join a yoga class later in the week. Trying new forms of exercise can also introduce you to new social circles, making it a great way to stay connected with others while staying active.

5. Listen to Your Body

Above all, Coach Elena Ruiz emphasizes the importance of listening to your body's signals. "Some days, you might feel strong and ready to push yourself, while other days, you might need to take it easy—and that's okay," she says. Recognizing when you need to rest or modify an exercise can help prevent burnout and injury.

Ruiz advises paying attention to any pain or discomfort, especially in the joints. "Pain is your body's way of telling you something isn't right. It's better to modify an exercise or take a break than to push through and risk a more serious injury," she explains. Rest days are an important part of any fitness routine, allowing muscles time to repair and grow stronger.

Building a Routine That Works for You

These expert tips can help guide you in creating a fitness routine that feels both effective and enjoyable. Remember, the goal is to stay active in a way that supports your health and fits into your life. In the final section, we'll explore how to make exercise a social activity, turning workouts into a fun and engaging part of your week.

Exercise as a Social Activity

Exercise doesn't have to be a solitary experience. In fact, turning workouts into a social activity can add a layer of enjoyment and motivation to your fitness routine. Exercising with friends or joining group activities not only makes staying active more fun but also provides an opportunity to build connections and a sense of community. Here are some ways to make exercise a social activity and enjoy the benefits of moving together.

1. Join a Walking Group or Club

Walking is one of the most accessible forms of exercise, and it's even better when shared with others. Many communities have walking groups or clubs that meet regularly, offering a chance to explore local parks and trails while getting in some cardio. Walking with a group can make the time pass more quickly and turn exercise into a social event.

If you can't find a local walking group, consider starting one with friends or neighbors. You can set a regular time each week to meet up and walk together, creating a routine that everyone looks forward to. It's a great way to catch up, enjoy the outdoors, and stay active all at once.

2. Try Group Fitness Classes

Group fitness classes can be a fun way to try new types of exercise and meet like-minded people. Many gyms, community centers, and even local parks offer classes tailored for different fitness levels. Whether it's yoga, Pilates, Zumba, or aqua aerobics, these classes provide a structured workout led by an instructor who can guide you through each movement.

One of the benefits of group classes is the sense of accountability they create. When you know others are expecting you to show up, it can be a great motivator to stick to your exercise routine. Plus, having an instructor ensures that you're using proper form, which can help prevent injuries and make the most of your workout.

3. Find an Exercise Buddy

Having a workout partner can make a big difference in staying consistent with your fitness routine. An exercise buddy can be a friend, family member, or neighbor who shares similar fitness goals. You can encourage each other on tough days and celebrate progress together. Even if you don't do the same workouts, simply agreeing to meet at the gym or go for a walk at the same time can add an element of social support.

Exercise buddies can also make activities like hiking, cycling, or taking a fitness class more enjoyable. Sharing the experience can turn what might feel like a chore into an opportunity for connection. Plus, a little friendly competition can push you to work harder and achieve new fitness milestones.

4. Participate in Community Events

Many communities host events like charity walks, 5K runs, or outdoor yoga sessions. These events are often open to participants of all ages and fitness levels, making them a great way to be active while supporting a good cause. Participating in a community event can give you a goal to work toward, like training for a local walk or run, and offer a sense of accomplishment when you complete it.

Charity events can add a sense of purpose to your exercise routine. Knowing that your efforts are contributing to a meaningful cause can make the experience more rewarding.

Plus, these events often include a festive atmosphere with music and food, and the chance to meet new people who share your interests.

5. Virtual Workouts: Staying Connected from Afar
For those who prefer to exercise at home or have friends and family living far away, virtual workouts can be a great way to stay connected. Many fitness apps and streaming platforms offer live classes that you can join with friends, or you can set up a virtual workout session via video chat. This allows you to exercise together, even when you're not in the same place.

Virtual workouts are also a convenient option for those with busy schedules, as you can fit them in whenever it works best for you. It's as simple as logging on to a Zoom or FaceTime call with a friend and doing a yoga flow or strength training routine together. This way, you can maintain the social aspect of exercising even when circumstances make it difficult to meet in person.

The Power of Community in Fitness
Making exercise a social activity can provide motivation, accountability, and a sense of belonging that enriches your fitness journey. Whether you prefer walking with friends, attending classes, or participating in community events, being active together can make a positive impact on your physical and emotional well-being. In addition, the friendships you build along the way can become an important support system, encouraging you to keep moving forward. In the next chapter, we'll explore the benefits of mindfulness and how to cultivate a positive mindset to complement your active lifestyle.

Chapter 5: Mindfulness and Mental Wellness: Cultivating a Positive Mindset

The Importance of Mental Wellness

Mental wellness is an integral part of overall well-being, especially as we age. It encompasses everything from how we think and feel to how we handle stress, make decisions, and connect with others. For women over 50, maintaining mental wellness is not just about avoiding anxiety or depression—it's about cultivating a mindset that allows us to find joy, purpose, and fulfillment in each day. Understanding the importance of mental wellness and how it can positively impact every aspect of life is the first step toward embracing a more balanced and fulfilling life.

1. Mental Wellness and Physical Health

The connection between mental and physical health is well-documented. When we feel mentally well, it's easier to take care of our physical health, whether that means staying active, eating nutritious foods, or maintaining healthy sleep habits. Conversely, stress, anxiety, and depression can take a toll on the body, manifesting as headaches, digestive issues, and even a weakened immune system.

Chronic stress can be a major challenge as we age, affecting everything from heart health to cognitive function. It triggers the release of cortisol, a stress hormone that, when elevated for extended periods, can contribute to inflammation in the body. Finding ways to manage stress and prioritize mental wellness can help reduce these physical effects, supporting overall health and longevity.

2. Staying Connected and Building Relationships

Social connections play a significant role in mental wellness. As we get older, life changes like retirement, moving to a new location, or the loss of loved ones can impact on our social circles and leave us feeling isolated. Loneliness and social isolation have been linked to increased risks of depression and anxiety, making it more important than ever to nurture relationships and seek out new connections.

Staying connected with friends, family, and community groups can provide a sense of belonging and purpose. Volunteering, joining clubs, or participating in community events are all ways to meet new people and build meaningful relationships. These social interactions not only provide emotional support but also help stimulate the mind, keeping it engaged and active.

3. Embracing the Changes of Aging

Aging often comes with a mix of changes, from shifts in physical abilities to changes in family dynamics. For some, this can bring about feelings of loss or uncertainty about the future. It's natural to feel a sense of nostalgia for what once was, but it's equally important to find ways to embrace the present and look forward to new possibilities.

Embracing change is a key component of mental wellness. It means learning to accept the things we can't control and focusing on what we can influence, like our attitudes and choices. It also means being open to new experiences, even if they feel outside of our comfort zones. This openness can make it easier to adapt to life's transitions, turning challenges into opportunities for growth.

4. Seeking Help When Needed

Taking care of mental wellness doesn't mean doing it all alone. Sometimes, reaching out for support from a mental health professional can be a crucial part of the process. Therapy, counseling, or support groups can provide a safe space to talk through emotions, gain new perspectives, and develop coping strategies for managing stress and anxiety.

There's no shame in seeking help—just as we see a doctor for physical ailments, mental health care is a normal and healthy part of taking care of ourselves. Many people find that therapy becomes a valuable tool for navigating major life transitions, such as adjusting to an empty nest, coping with grief, or managing the stress that comes with aging.

5. Finding Joy in Everyday Moments

Mental wellness isn't just about managing challenges—it's also about finding joy in the simple pleasures of life. This might mean taking time each morning to savor a cup of tea, watching the sunset, or spending time with a beloved pet. Mindfulness practices, like focusing on the present moment and appreciating the small things, can help us become more aware of these joyful moments and make them a regular part of our day.

The more we practice finding joy in everyday moments, the easier it becomes to maintain a positive outlook, even when faced with difficulties. It's a way of training the mind to focus on the good rather than getting caught up in worries about the past or future. This doesn't mean ignoring challenges, but rather balancing them with a sense of gratitude and contentment.

The Path to Greater Well-being

Understanding the importance of mental wellness is a powerful starting point for living a balanced and joyful life.

By prioritizing social connections, embracing change, seeking support when needed, and finding joy in the present, we can build a mindset that allows us to thrive at any age. In the next section, we'll explore specific mindfulness practices that can bring calmer and focus to your everyday routine, helping you cultivate a greater sense of peace and well-being.

Mindfulness Practices for Everyday Calm

Mindfulness is the practice of being fully present in the moment, allowing yourself to experience life without distraction or judgment. It's about bringing attention to what's happening right now—whether it's the sound of the wind, the warmth of a cup of tea, or the rise and fall of your breath. For many women over 50, incorporating mindfulness practices into daily life can be a powerful way to reduce stress, improve focus, and cultivate a deeper sense of peace.

1. Mindful Breathing

One of the simplest ways to practice mindfulness is through mindful breathing. This technique can be done anywhere—while sitting at your desk, lying in bed, or even while waiting in line. It involves focusing your attention on your breath, noticing the sensation of air entering and leaving your body.

To practice, find a comfortable position and close your eyes if it feels right. Take a slow, deep breath in through your nose, feeling your chest and belly expand. Then, exhale slowly through your mouth, letting go of any tension. Try to keep your attention on the rhythm of your breath. If your mind starts to wander, gently guide it back to the sensation of breathing. Even a few minutes of mindful breathing each day can help calm the mind and reduce feelings of anxiety.

2. Body Scan Meditation

The body scan is another effective mindfulness practice that helps you reconnect with your body and release physical tension. It involves bringing awareness to different parts of your body, one at a time, and noticing any sensations without trying to change them. The body scan can be especially helpful for those who experience stress-related muscle tension or have trouble falling asleep.

To begin, lie down in a comfortable position or sit with your feet flat on the floor. Close your eyes and take a few deep breaths. Start by focusing on your toes, noticing any sensations there—warmth, coolness, tingling, or even a lack of sensation. Slowly move your attention up through your feet, ankles, legs, and continue all the way to the top of your head. As you focus on each area, try to release any tension you might be holding. This practice can be done in as little as five minutes or extended to a longer relaxation session.

3. Mindful Eating

Mindful eating is a practice that helps you fully enjoy and appreciate your meals. It involves slowing down and paying attention to the taste, texture, and aroma of your food, as well as your body's hunger and fullness cues. For many people, eating can become a rushed or distracting activity, but mindful eating transforms it into an opportunity for self-care.

To practice mindful eating, start by taking a moment to appreciate your food before you take your first bite. Notice the colors, the smell, and how the food looks on your plate. As you eat, try to chew slowly and savor each bite. Focus on the flavors and textures in your mouth and pause between bites to give your body time to register fullness. This practice not only enhances your enjoyment of food but can also improve digestion and prevent overeating.

4. Walking Meditation

For those who find it difficult to sit still, walking meditation can be a wonderful alternative. This practice combines the benefits of gentle movement with the focus of mindfulness. It's especially effective in a natural setting, like a park or garden, where you can tune into the sounds and sights around you.

To begin, find a quiet place where you can walk slowly without interruptions. Start by standing still for a moment and taking a few deep breaths. As you begin to walk, focus on the sensation of your feet touching the ground, the movement of your legs, and the rhythm of your steps. Notice the feeling of the air on your skin and the sounds around you. The goal is not to reach a destination but to fully experience the act of walking.

5. Gratitude Journaling

Keeping a gratitude journal is a simple yet powerful mindfulness practice that can shift your focus from what's lacking in life to what's abundant. Each day, take a few minutes to write down three things you're grateful for. These can be big things, like good health or a supportive friend, or small moments, like a beautiful sunrise or a warm cup of tea.

The act of writing down what you're grateful for helps train your mind to notice the positive aspects of life. Over time, this practice can increase feelings of contentment and reduce stress. Many people find that writing in their gratitude journal at night helps them end the day on a positive note, making it easier to relax and sleep well.

Creating a Mindfulness Routine
Mindfulness practices don't have to take a lot of time, and they don't require any special equipment. By incorporating just one or two of these practices into your daily routine, you can create a sense of calm and balance that supports your overall mental wellness. In the next section, we'll explore how building resilience and embracing change can further enhance your journey toward a positive mindset.

Building Resilience and Embracing Change

Life is full of transitions, and as we age, these changes can come with new challenges, from shifts in physical health to evolving roles within our families and communities. Building resilience—our ability to adapt and thrive in the face of adversity—is key to navigating these changes with a positive mindset. Resilience doesn't mean avoiding difficulties; rather, it's about facing them with strength, adaptability, and a belief in our ability to move forward.

1. Acknowledge and Accept Change
One of the first steps to building resilience is learning to acknowledge and accept change as a natural part of life. Resistance to change can create stress and frustration, while acceptance allows us to adapt more smoothly. This doesn't mean that all changes are easy or welcome retirement, the loss of a loved one, or adjusting to new physical limitations can be challenging. However, accepting that change is a part of life helps us focus our energy on finding solutions rather than dwelling on what's beyond our control.

Mindfulness can play a role here, helping us stay grounded in the present rather than worrying about the past or future. By focusing on what we can do in the moment, we can gradually adjust to new realities, finding a sense of peace even when life takes unexpected turns.

2. Cultivate a Growth Mindset

A growth mindset—the belief that abilities and intelligence can be developed over time—can be a powerful tool for building resilience. This mindset encourages us to see challenges not as setbacks but as opportunities for growth. Psychologist Carol Dweck, who pioneered the concept, emphasizes that a growth mindset allows us to persist through difficulties, learn new skills, and find new ways to overcome obstacles.

For example, if physical limitations make a favorite activity more challenging, a growth mindset might encourage you to explore a modified version of that activity or to try something entirely new. Instead of focusing on what's no longer possible, it shifts the focus to what you can achieve with the resources available to you. Embracing this perspective can make the journey of aging feel like a time of continued learning and exploration, rather than a period of decline.

3. Build a Support System

Having a strong support system is essential for resilience. Friends, family, and community connections provide a sense of belonging and a source of encouragement during difficult times. When facing challenges, having people to talk to can help us process emotions and gain perspective. Social support has been shown to improve mental health, reduce feelings of isolation, and even increase longevity.

Building a support system doesn't have to be complicated. It can be as simple as reaching out to a friend for coffee, joining a local club or volunteer group, or attending social events in your community. The goal is to find people who uplift you and make you feel heard and valued. In turn, offering support to others can be just as rewarding, creating a cycle of mutual encouragement that strengthens everyone involved.

4. Practice Self-Compassion

Resilience is not about being tough all the time—it's also about being kind to yourself when things are difficult. Self-compassion involves treating yourself with the same understanding and care that you would offer to a close friend. When you experience setbacks or feel overwhelmed, it's important to recognize that these feelings are a normal part of being human, especially during times of transition.

Practicing self-compassion might mean giving yourself permission to rest when you're feeling tired or allowing yourself to feel sad without judgment. It's about acknowledging your feelings without being too harsh on yourself. Studies have shown that self-compassion can help reduce anxiety and depression, making it easier to cope with life's challenges.

5. Focus on What You Can Control

In any situation, it's helpful to distinguish between what you can control and what you cannot. Focusing on what's within your control can prevent feelings of helplessness and empower you to take positive action. For example, while we can't control the aging process, we can choose how we take care of our bodies, manage our time, and engage with our communities.

Making a list of the things you can control in a difficult situation can be a practical way to shift your focus. It might include actions like maintaining a healthy diet, reaching out to friends, or setting small, achievable goals. By concentrating on these areas, you can create a sense of purpose and direction, even during challenging times.

Finding Strength in Change
Building resilience is a lifelong journey, and it's a skill that can be strengthened at any age. By embracing change, seeking support, practicing self-compassion, and focusing on growth, you can navigate life's transitions with greater ease and confidence. In the next section, we'll explore how gratitude and positive thinking can further enhance your mental well-being, helping you find joy and meaning in everyday life.

The Role of Gratitude and Positive Thinking

Gratitude and positive thinking are powerful tools for enhancing mental wellness. They help shift our focus from what's lacking in life to the abundance that surrounds us, even in the midst of challenges. For many women over 50, cultivating a mindset of gratitude can provide a sense of peace and joy, helping to navigate life's transitions with a lighter heart. Here's how practicing gratitude and positive thinking can positively impact your well-being and how to incorporate these practices into your daily life.

1. The Science Behind Gratitude
Gratitude isn't just a feel-good concept; it's backed by scientific research. Studies have shown that practicing gratitude can increase overall happiness, improve sleep, and even boost the immune system. When we express

gratitude, the brain releases dopamine and serotonin—chemicals that enhance mood and make us feel good. Over time, this can help rewire the brain to focus more on positive experiences, making it easier to maintain a sunny outlook.

Gratitude also helps to reduce stress. When we focus on the things we're thankful for, it's harder for worries to take center stage. This doesn't mean ignoring challenges, but rather balancing them with an awareness of the good in our lives. For example, while adjusting to physical changes might be difficult, a focus on gratitude could highlight the support of loved ones or the beauty of a peaceful walk in nature.

2. Keeping a Gratitude Journal

One of the most effective ways to practice gratitude is by keeping a gratitude journal. This involves taking a few minutes each day to write down things you're grateful for. These entries can be as simple as a delicious cup of coffee in the morning or as meaningful as a deep conversation with a friend.

Many people find that writing in their gratitude journal before bed helps them end the day on a positive note, making it easier to let go of stress and enjoy restful sleep. Over time, this habit can become a source of comfort and a reminder of the positive aspects of life, even during challenging times. It's a simple practice that doesn't take much time but can have a profound impact on your mindset.

3. Positive Affirmations for a Brighter Mindset

Positive affirmations are short, powerful statements that can help shift your thinking patterns. They are designed to counter negative thoughts and reinforce a more positive self-image. For example, repeating affirmations like "I am strong and capable" or "I embrace each day with gratitude and joy" can help build confidence and resilience.

To practice, choose a few affirmations that resonate with you and repeat them daily, either out loud or in your mind. You might say them in front of a mirror in the morning, write them in your journal, or use them as a focus during meditation. The key is to use affirmations that feel authentic and meaningful to you. Over time, these positive statements can help reshape your inner dialogue, making it easier to face challenges with a hopeful attitude.

4. Reframing Negative Thoughts

Positive thinking isn't about ignoring the difficulties in life; it's about learning to reframe negative thoughts in a way that empowers you. When faced with a setback, instead of thinking "I can't handle this," try shifting the thought to "This is difficult, but I have overcome challenges before, and I can find a way through this one too." This shift in perspective can help you approach problems with a solution-oriented mindset.

Reframing is a skill that takes practice, but it can be transformative. It allows you to see obstacles as opportunities for growth rather than insurmountable barriers. This doesn't mean you have to force yourself to be positive all the time, but rather that you acknowledge your feelings and choose to focus on what you can do to improve the situation.

5. Gratitude in Action

Expressing gratitude doesn't have to be limited to private reflections; it can also be a powerful way to connect with others. Taking the time to thank a friend, writing a note of appreciation, or express gratitude to a loved one can strengthen relationships and spread positivity. Acts of kindness, such as volunteering or helping a neighbor, can also be an expression of gratitude, allowing you to share your appreciation for the world around you.

For many people, these actions bring a sense of fulfillment and purpose. They remind us that we are part of a larger community, and that our efforts to spread kindness and gratitude can make a meaningful difference. In return, these connections can provide support and comfort, especially during times when you might need it most.

A Daily Practice for a Brighter Outlook
Incorporating gratitude and positive thinking into your daily life can transform the way you experience the world. It's a practice that can bring more joy into everyday moments, help you weather difficult times with grace, and foster a deeper appreciation for the life you're living. In the next section, we'll explore self-care rituals that support emotional well-being, offering practical ways to nurture your mind and spirit.

Self-Care Rituals for Emotional Well-being

Self-care is about more than just pampering yourself—it's an essential practice for maintaining emotional well-being, especially during times of change or stress. For women over 50, self-care can take many forms, from small daily rituals that bring joy to more intentional practices that nurture the mind and spirit. Here's how to create self-care routines that support your emotional health and bring a sense of balance to your life.

1. Morning Rituals for a Positive Start

Starting your day with a mindful morning routine can set a positive tone for the hours ahead. This might include simple activities like stretching, enjoying a warm cup of herbal tea, or spending a few minutes journaling your thoughts and intentions for the day. For many, taking time to practice gratitude or recite positive affirmations in the morning can help cultivate a sense of optimism.

Mindful mornings don't have to be elaborate. Even setting aside 10-15 minutes to focus on yourself before diving into the day's responsibilities can make a significant difference. The goal is to create a ritual that feels grounding and helps you feel centered, so that you can approach the day with a clear mind and an open heart.

2. Creating a Relaxing Evening Routine

Just as mornings are a time for setting intentions, evenings are an opportunity to wind down and let go of the day's stresses. An evening routine that helps you relax and prepare for restful sleep can improve both your physical and emotional health. This might include activities like reading a book, taking a warm bath with calming essential oils like lavender, or practicing gentle stretches to release muscle tension.

Some people find that turning off screens at least an hour before bed and opting for a calming activity, like listening to soft music or meditating, can help signal to the body that it's time to rest. Consistency is key—by following the same routine each night, you can create a comforting end to your day that promotes deeper, more restorative sleep.

3. Nature Walks for Mindfulness and Connection

Spending time in nature is a simple yet powerful way to practice self-care. Nature has a calming effect on the mind, helping to reduce anxiety and promote a sense of peace. A leisurely walk in a local park or by the beach can provide a chance to disconnect from technology and reconnect with yourself.

Nature walks can be an opportunity for mindful walking, where you focus on the sights, sounds, and smells around you, letting go of any worries or to-do lists. This practice can help ground you in the present moment, providing a mental reset. Even a short 10–20-minute walk outside can make a big difference in how you feel throughout the day.

4. Creative Expression as Self-Care
Engaging in creative activities can be a wonderful way to express yourself and process your emotions. Whether it's painting, knitting, writing, or playing an instrument, creative expression allows you to explore your inner world and find joy in the act of creating something new. It's a form of self-care that provides a break from routine and offers a sense of accomplishment.

For those who may not consider themselves "artistic," it's important to remember that the goal is not perfection but enjoyment. Allow yourself to experiment without judgment and embrace the process of trying new things. Joining a local art class or creative workshop can also be a great way to meet new people and share your creative journey with others.

5. Treating Yourself with Kindness
Self-care is ultimately about treating yourself with kindness and compassion. It means listening to your body and mind and recognizing when you need a break. This might mean taking a day off from your usual routine, giving yourself permission to rest, or enjoying a special treat without guilt.

Sometimes, self-care can be as simple as setting boundaries and learning to say no when you feel overwhelmed. It's about prioritizing your own needs and recognizing that it's okay to take time for yourself. This is especially important for those who have spent years focusing on the needs of others—self-care is a reminder that your well-being matters, too.

Making Self-Care a Priority
By incorporating self-care rituals into your daily routine, you can create a space for healing, reflection, and renewal. These practices are not just about reducing stress, they're about finding ways to connect with yourself and rediscover what makes you feel most alive. In the next chapter, we'll explore how to adapt to physical changes with grace, embracing the beauty of each stage of life with confidence and self-love.

Chapter 6: Adapting to Physical Changes: Accepting and Adjusting with Grace

Understanding Physical Changes

Aging is a natural part of life, and with it comes a range of physical changes that can feel both challenging and transformative. Understanding these changes can make it easier to adapt to them with grace and confidence, allowing you to continue feeling comfortable in your own body. While some changes might be more noticeable than others, learning about what to expect can help you approach this stage of life with a sense of acceptance and self-compassion.

1. Changes in Skin and Hair
One of the most visible changes as we age is the transformation of our skin and hair. Skin naturally becomes thinner and loses elasticity over time, leading to the appearance of fine lines, wrinkles, and a more delicate texture. This is due in part to a decrease in collagen and elastin production, proteins that keep skin firm and resilient. While these changes are a normal part of aging, there are ways to support your skin's health through a gentle skincare routine and by staying hydrated.

Hair also undergoes changes with age, often becoming finer, thinner, and more prone to dryness. Graying hair is another natural sign of aging, as the pigment-producing cells in hair follicles gradually reduce their activity. While some choose to embrace their natural gray, others may prefer to maintain their original color with gentle hair dye. Whichever choice feels right for you, it's important to use products that nourish and protect your hair, especially as it becomes more sensitive to chemical treatments.

2. Shifts in Metabolism and Weight

Metabolism tends to slow down as we age, which can make it more challenging to maintain a stable weight. Hormonal changes, particularly around menopause, can also affect body composition, leading to a redistribution of weight around the midsection. This can be a source of frustration for many women, but it's important to remember that these changes are a normal part of the aging process.

A slower metabolism means that the body burns fewer calories at rest, making it easier to gain weight if eating habits remain the same. Adjusting your diet to focus on nutrient-dense foods, such as lean proteins, whole grains, and plenty of fruits and vegetables, can help support a healthy metabolism. Pairing this with regular physical activity, including both cardio and strength training, can help maintain muscle mass and support overall metabolic health.

3. Bone Density and Joint Health

Bone density naturally decreases with age, especially in women after menopause, due to a drop in estrogen levels. This loss of bone mass can increase the risk of osteoporosis, a condition that makes bones more fragile and susceptible to fractures. Keeping bones strong requires a combination of weight-bearing exercises, like walking or resistance training, and a diet rich in calcium and vitamin D to support bone health.

Joint health can also become more of a concern as we age, with many people experiencing stiffness, discomfort, or conditions like arthritis. Staying active with low-impact exercises, such as swimming, yoga, or tai chi, can help maintain flexibility and reduce stiffness in the joints. It's also important to listen to your body's signals and make adjustments as needed, such as using supportive footwear or taking breaks during activities.

4. Changes in Vision and Hearing
Changes in vision and hearing are common as we age. Many people find that they need reading glasses or have difficulty seeing them in low light as they get older. This is often due to a natural stiffening of the eye's lens, which makes it harder to focus on close objects. Regular eye exams are important for monitoring changes in vision and ensuring that any necessary adjustments, like updated prescriptions, are made.

Hearing changes can also occur gradually, with many people noticing that certain frequencies become harder to hear. This can make it difficult to follow conversations in noisy environments or understand higher-pitched sounds. Hearing aids and assistive devices can be a valuable support, allowing you to continue enjoying social interactions and staying connected with others.

5. Embracing a New Perspective
Understanding these physical changes can help you approach them with greater acceptance. While it's natural to wish for the energy and appearance of younger years, it's also important to recognize the wisdom and strength that come with age. Embracing this perspective allows you to focus on what your body can do, rather than what it can no longer do. This shift in mindset can turn aging into an opportunity for self-discovery and growth, making it easier to navigate physical changes with grace and confidence.

In the next section, we'll explore how to stay active while adapting to these changes, helping you maintain mobility and strength as you continue to enjoy life to the fullest.

Staying Active While Adjusting

Staying active is one of the best ways to support your health and well-being as you navigate the physical changes that come with aging. While these changes may require you to adjust your exercise routine, they don't mean you have to slow down or give up the activities you love. Adapting your approach to fitness can help you maintain strength, flexibility, and energy levels, allowing you to continue enjoying a full and active life. Here are some tips for staying active while adjusting to your body's evolving needs.

1. Listen to Your Body

As we age, it's important to pay closer attention to what our bodies are telling us. This means being mindful of any aches, pains, or signs of fatigue and adjusting when necessary. Pushing through discomfort can lead to injuries, which are more difficult to recover from later in life. Instead, focus on finding a balance between challenging yourself and respecting your body's limits.

This might mean swapping high-impact activities like running for lower-impact alternatives such as walking, swimming, or cycling. It could also mean incorporating more rest days into your routine to allow your muscles and joints time to recover. By listening to your body and adjusting your activities as needed, you can stay active without overexertion.

2. Focus on Mobility and Flexibility

Maintaining mobility and flexibility is essential for everyday activities, from reaching for items on a high shelf to bending down to tie your shoes. As we age, muscles and joints can become stiffer, making it harder to move freely. Incorporating stretching exercises into your routine can help keep your body limber and reduce the risk of injury.

Yoga and Pilates are excellent options for improving flexibility while also strengthening core muscles. These practices focus on controlled movements and deep stretching, which can help ease tension in the body. Even simple daily stretches, like reaching for your toes or stretching your arms overhead, can make a big difference in maintaining range of motion and preventing stiffness.

3. Strength Training for Functional Fitness

Strength training becomes even more important as we age, as it helps to counteract the natural loss of muscle mass and supports bone density. However, the way we approach strength training may need to change. Lifting lighter weights with more repetitions can be just as effective as heavier lifting and is often easier on the joints. Resistance bands are another great option for adding gentle resistance without the need for heavy equipment.

Focus on functional fitness exercises that mimic everyday movements and help you maintain the strength needed for daily tasks. For example, squats can make it easier to get in and out of chairs, while modified push-ups can help build the upper body strength needed to carry groceries. Aiming for two to three strength training sessions per week can help maintain muscle tone and support overall mobility.

4. Keep It Low-Impact

Low-impact exercises are gentle on the joints while still

providing a great workout for the heart and muscles. Activities like swimming, water aerobics, walking, and using an elliptical machine offer the benefits of cardiovascular exercise without the jarring impact that running or jumping can have on the knees and hips.

Swimming is a favorite for many older adults because the buoyancy of the water supports the body, reducing strain on the joints while still offering resistance that builds muscle. Water-based exercises are also ideal for those with arthritis or chronic pain, as they allow you to stay active without aggravating sensitive areas.

5. Adapt Your Routine as Needed
Your exercise routine should evolve with you, adapting to your changing needs and goals. This might mean trying new activities that you've never considered before, like tai chi, which combines gentle movement with deep breathing and mindfulness. It could also mean modifying exercises to suit your current abilities—using a chair for support during balance exercises, for example, or opting for shorter workout sessions that you can do consistently.

Remember, the goal is not to compete with younger versions of yourself, but to find ways to stay active that feel good and keep you engaged. By focusing on consistency rather than intensity, you can build a sustainable routine that keeps you strong and active for years to come.

Finding Joy in Movement
Staying active is about more than just maintaining physical health—it's also about finding joy in movement and embracing activities that make you feel good. Whether it's a walk in the park, a gentle yoga class, or a new hobby like gardening or dance, staying active can be a source of pleasure and connection. In the next section, we'll explore

common health concerns and how to manage them effectively, ensuring that you continue to feel your best while adapting to life's changes.

Managing Common Health Concerns

As we age, certain health concerns become more common, but with the right knowledge and proactive management, many of these conditions can be addressed effectively. Staying informed and working closely with healthcare providers can help you maintain your quality of life while managing changes in your body. Here's a look at some of the most common health concerns for women over 50 and how to manage them.

1. Bone Health and Osteoporosis

Osteoporosis, a condition where bones become brittle and fragile due to loss of density, is particularly common among postmenopausal women. The decrease in estrogen levels after menopause can accelerate bone loss, increasing the risk of fractures, especially in the spine, hips, and wrists. Regular weight-bearing exercises like walking, hiking, or resistance training can help strengthen bones, while stretching and balance exercises like yoga can reduce the risk of falls.

A diet rich in calcium and vitamin D is also crucial for maintaining bone health. Calcium helps build and maintain strong bones, while vitamin D improves calcium absorption. Foods like dairy products, leafy greens, and fortified cereals are excellent sources of calcium. Sun exposure can help the body produce vitamin D, but supplements might be necessary for those living in less sunny climates or who have difficulty absorbing the nutrient. Discussing bone density screenings with your healthcare provider can help you monitor your bone health and adjust your diet or exercise routine as needed.

2. Heart Health

Heart disease is one of the leading health concerns for women over 50. As metabolism slows down and estrogen levels decline, changes in cholesterol levels and blood pressure can increase the risk of cardiovascular issues. Maintaining a heart-healthy lifestyle through diet, exercise, and stress management is key to reducing these risks.

Focus on a diet that includes plenty of fruits, vegetables, whole grains, and healthy fats like those found in nuts, seeds, and olive oil. Reducing sodium intake and avoiding processed foods can help manage blood pressure. Aerobic activities like walking, swimming, or dancing can strengthen the heart and improve circulation. It's also important to manage stress, as chronic stress can contribute to high blood pressure. Practices like meditation, deep breathing, and spending time in nature can help keep stress levels in check.

3. Joint Health and Arthritis

Arthritis, particularly osteoarthritis, is common as we age, affecting joints like the knees, hips, and hands. It can cause pain, stiffness, and swelling, making it harder to stay active. However, movement is one of the best ways to manage arthritis symptoms, as it helps keep joints flexible and strengthens the muscles that support them.

Low-impact exercises like swimming, water aerobics, and cycling are particularly beneficial, as they provide a full-body workout without putting excess strain on the joints. Strength training can also help by building the muscles around the affected joints, providing better support and

reducing pain. Stretching exercises and yoga can improve
flexibility and alleviate stiffness. For those experiencing
significant discomfort, physical therapy can provide
tailored exercises and strategies to improve mobility.

4. Menopause and Hormonal Changes
Menopause brings a range of changes, from hot flashes and
night sweats to mood swings and changes in weight
distribution. While menopause is a natural transition, its
symptoms can impact quality of life. Managing these
symptoms often requires a combination of lifestyle
adjustments, natural remedies, and, in some cases, medical
support.

For hot flashes and night sweats, dressing in layers,
keeping the bedroom cool, and using a fan can provide
relief. Some women find that natural supplements like
black cohosh or evening primrose oil help with menopausal
symptoms, though it's important to consult with a
healthcare provider before starting any new supplements.
Hormone replacement therapy (HRT) can also be an option
for managing more severe symptoms, but it should be
discussed with a doctor to weigh the potential benefits and
risks.

5. Maintaining Mental Health
Mental health is just as important as physical health, and
many women over 50 face challenges like anxiety,
depression, or feelings of isolation. Hormonal changes can
affect mood, while life transitions such as retirement,
becoming an empty nester, or experiencing the loss of
loved ones can bring emotional stress.

Staying socially connected is one of the best ways to
support mental health. Joining local clubs, taking up a
hobby, or participating in volunteer work can provide

opportunities for new friendships and a sense of purpose. Regular exercise also boosts endorphins, helping to reduce symptoms of anxiety and depression. In cases where feelings of sadness or anxiety persist, seeking support from a therapist or counselor can be a valuable step. Therapy provides a space to talk through feelings, learn coping strategies, and find new ways to adapt to life's changes.

Taking Control of Your Health
Managing these common health concerns requires a proactive approach, but the effort is well worth it for maintaining independence and quality of life. Regular check-ups with your healthcare provider, a balanced diet, and an active lifestyle all contribute to feeling your best as you navigate the changes that come with aging. In the next section, we'll explore how to adapt your beauty and style routine to complement these changes, helping you feel confident and vibrant at any age.

Adapting Your Beauty and Style Routine

As we age, our sense of style and the way we approach beauty can evolve, just as our bodies do. Rather than trying to maintain the same routines from years past, adapting your beauty and style to meet your current needs can be a powerful way to celebrate this stage of life. By embracing new techniques, products, and fashion choices, you can highlight your best features and feel confident at any age. Here's how to refresh your beauty and style routine to match the changes that come with aging.

1. Skincare That Embraces Change
With age, skin tends to become drier and more sensitive, making it important to choose skincare products that

hydrate and nourish without irritating. Consider switching to a richer moisturizer that includes ingredients like hyaluronic acid, ceramides, and peptides, which help to lock in moisture and support skin elasticity. Gentle cleansers that don't strip the skin of natural oils can also help maintain a healthy barrier, keeping your skin feeling soft and hydrated.

Incorporating a serum with antioxidants, like vitamin C, can brighten the complexion and help protect against environmental damage. Retinol, a derivative of vitamin A, can be particularly effective for reducing the appearance of fine lines and promoting smoother skin texture. If you're new to retinol, start with a low-strength product and use it a few times a week to avoid irritation.

2. Makeup Tips for Mature Skin

Makeup can be a wonderful way to enhance your natural beauty, but the techniques that worked in your 30s and 40s may need a few adjustments as your skin changes. As skin becomes thinner and more prone to dryness, opting for lightweight, hydrating formulas can help avoid a cakey or overly matte look. A tinted moisturizer or a lightweight foundation can provide a fresh, dewy finish while evening out skin tone.

For the eye area, cream-based eyeshadows are often more flattering than powders, as they are less likely to settle into fine lines. Using a gentle touch when applying eyeliner and choosing softer shades like brown or gray can create a more natural look. Blush and highlighter can add a healthy glow to the cheeks—cream blushes are particularly flattering on mature skin, giving a youthful flush that blends seamlessly.

3. Haircare That Reflects Your Style

Hair texture and thickness often change with age, but that

doesn't mean your hair can't look fabulous. Choosing products that add moisture, and volume can make a big difference in how your hair looks and feels. Consider using a hydrating shampoo and conditioner and add a lightweight styling cream or serum to tame frizz and add shine.

If you're embracing your natural gray, a purple shampoo can help neutralize any yellow tones and keep your silver strands looking vibrant. For those who prefer to maintain their original color, switching to gentler hair dyes and avoiding excessive heat styling can protect hair health. No matter your hair color, a flattering cut that suits your face shape can instantly refresh your look. Many stylists recommend shorter cuts or adding layers to create movement and add fullness.

4. Fashion That Fits Your Personality

Fashion is a powerful way to express who you are, and there's no age limit on dressing with style and confidence. As we get older, it's normal to gravitate toward clothes that offer comfort and practicality, but this doesn't mean sacrificing style. Investing in well-fitting basics like tailored pants, comfortable yet stylish shoes, and soft, breathable fabrics can create a versatile wardrobe that looks polished without feeling restrictive.

Accessories can also play a key role in adding flair to your outfits. Scarves, statement jewelry, and hats can elevate even the simplest looks, adding a touch of personality. Many women find that they enjoy experimenting with bolder colors and prints as they age, using fashion as a way to express their individuality.

5. Embracing Your Unique Beauty

Above all, the most important part of any beauty or style routine is feeling comfortable in your own skin. While products and techniques can help you look and feel your best, true beauty comes from embracing who you are at every stage of life. This means letting go of unrealistic expectations and focusing on what makes you feel confident and happy.

Take time to celebrate the features you love about yourself—whether it's your smile, your eyes, or the unique style you've cultivated over the years. Confidence is the ultimate accessory, and embracing your own unique beauty is the best way to let it shine. Aging is a privilege, and adapting your beauty and style routines is a way to honor the journey you've been on.

Style with Confidence
Adapting your beauty and style routine to match the changes in your body is about celebrating the person you are today. By choosing skincare, makeup, haircare, and fashion that enhance your natural features and reflect your personality, you can continue to feel vibrant and stylish at every age. In the next section, we'll explore how to embrace your changing body with self-love and acceptance, creating a positive and empowered outlook on aging.

Embracing Your Changing Body

Aging brings about many physical changes, but learning to embrace your body as it evolves is a powerful way to maintain a positive outlook and a sense of self-love. It's normal to feel a sense of loss when certain aspects of your appearance or physical abilities change, but it's also possible to shift your perspective and celebrate the strength and resilience of your body. Here's how to cultivate a mindset that embraces these changes with grace and confidence.

1. Letting Go of Unrealistic Standards

For many women, aging can bring a sense of pressure to maintain youthful looks, influenced by societal standards that often celebrate youth over experience. Letting go of these unrealistic standards is an important step in embracing your changing body. It means recognizing that beauty doesn't have an expiration date, and that confidence comes from accepting yourself as you are.

Consider shifting your focus from what your body used to look like to what it can do now. Instead of seeing wrinkles or gray hair as flaws, try to view them as symbols of a life well-lived—each line representing a laugh, a tear, or a moment of growth. By redefining beauty on your own terms, you can free yourself from the pressure of comparison and appreciate the uniqueness of your journey.

2. Practicing Self-Compassion

Self-compassion involves treating yourself with the same kindness and understanding that you would offer a close friend. It means being gentle with yourself on days when you feel self-critical or frustrated by physical changes. Practicing self-compassion allows you to acknowledge those feelings without letting them define how you see yourself.

One way to practice self-compassion is through positive self-talk. When you notice negative thoughts creeping in, try to counter them with affirming statements like "My body is strong and capable" or "I deserve love and care, just as I am." This shift in inner dialogue can make a big difference in how you feel about yourself, helping you build a more loving relationship with your body.

3. Celebrating What Your Body Can Do

Your body has carried you through many stages of life—through challenges, joys, and countless experiences that have shaped who you are today. Taking time to appreciate the strength and resilience of your body can shift your perspective from what you feel is lacking to what you have gained. For example, consider the strength it takes to walk, to hug loved ones, or to pursue new hobbies.

Celebrating what your body can do might mean finding joy in movement, whether it's through a daily walk, a dance class, or gardening. It could also involve trying new activities that challenge your body in new ways, like learning to swim or taking up yoga. By focusing on the capabilities of your body, you can create a sense of gratitude that deepens your appreciation for all it has done for you.

4. Dressing for Confidence and Comfort

Clothing is a powerful way to express yourself and choosing outfits that make you feel good can boost your confidence. As your body changes, you may find that different cuts, fabrics, or styles feel better than what you used to wear. The goal is not to hide your body but to find clothes that make you feel comfortable and confident.

Consider experimenting with new colors, patterns, and styles that reflect your personality and current tastes. Don't be afraid to step outside of your comfort zones sometimes a bold new piece can make you feel like you're embracing a new chapter of life. Remember, fashion is about self-expression, and dressing in a way that makes you feel beautiful is a form of self-care.

5. Connecting with a Community

It's easier to embrace change when you know you're not alone. Connecting with others who are going through similar experiences can provide support, encouragement, and a sense of solidarity. Joining groups or forums for women navigating midlife, participating in local activities, or even sharing your journey with friends can create a network of support.

Hearing the stories of other women who are learning to love their changing bodies can be incredibly empowering. It's a reminder that every woman's experience is unique, and there's no right or wrong way to feel about aging. Sharing your own experiences, too, can be a way to inspire others, creating a ripple effect of positivity and acceptance.

Embracing the Journey

Embracing your changing body is about honoring the past, celebrating the present, and looking forward to the future with openness and self-love. By letting go of unrealistic standards, practicing self-compassion, and focusing on what makes you feel good, you can create a more positive and empowered relationship with your body. The journey of aging is one of growth, and embracing it fully allows you to step into each new stage of life with grace and confidence. In the next chapter, we'll explore how to nurture your relationships and continue building a meaningful social life as you age.

Chapter 7: Nurturing Relationships: Building Connections and Community

The Importance of Social Connections

Maintaining strong social connections is one of the most important aspects of well-being as we age. Relationships provide a sense of belonging, offer emotional support, and help us stay engaged with the world around us. For women over 50, nurturing friendships and building community can make a significant difference in how we experience this stage of life, contributing to both mental and physical health. Understanding the importance of social connections can help you prioritize these bonds and create a fulfilling social life.

1. The Health Benefits of Staying Connected

Strong social ties have been shown to positively impact physical health. Studies suggest that people who maintain active social lives have lower risks of conditions like heart disease, high blood pressure, and cognitive decline. Engaging in social activities can help reduce stress, boost the immune system, and even contribute to a longer life.

On the emotional side, being connected to others provides a buffer against feelings of loneliness and isolation, which can become more common as we age. Loneliness has been linked to increased risks of depression and anxiety, but having a strong support network can provide a sense of security and companionship. It's not about the quantity of relationships but the quality—meaningful connections that provide mutual support and understanding are what matter most.

2. Emotional Support During Life Transitions
Life after 50 often comes with transitions, such as retirement, children leaving home, or the loss of a spouse or close friends. These changes can bring about feelings of loss or uncertainty, making social support even more important. Having people to share these experiences with can help ease the emotional burden and provide new perspectives on how to navigate change.

Friends and family can be a source of comfort during difficult times, offering a listening ear or simply being present. Sharing stories, laughter, and experiences helps us remember that we are not alone in our challenges. Sometimes, just knowing that someone is there for you can make all the difference in coping with life's ups and downs.

3. Staying Mentally Active Through Social Engagement
Engaging with others is not only good for the heart but also for the mind. Social interactions stimulate the brain, keeping it active and engaged. Whether it's through lively conversations, playing games, or learning new activities together, interacting with others helps keep cognitive skills sharp. This is especially important as we age, as maintaining mental activity can help reduce the risk of cognitive decline.

Participating in group activities, such as book clubs, art classes, or hobby groups, can provide opportunities to learn new things and challenge your mind. These activities often come with the added benefit of meeting new people who share similar interests, making it easier to expand your social circle.

4. Finding Joy in Shared Activities

Shared activities are a great way to deepen existing relationships and create new ones. Whether walking with a friend, joining a dance class, or volunteering for a local charity, doing things with others can make every day experiences more enjoyable. Shared activities provide a chance to bond over common interests and create lasting memories together.

For many women, these moments of connection become the highlights of the week—a time to laugh, share stories, and simply enjoy each other's company. Making time for these activities can provide a sense of routine and stability, which is especially valuable during times of change. It's a reminder that there's always something to look forward to, even when life feels uncertain.

5. Staying Connected in a Digital World

In today's digital age, technology has made it easier to stay connected with loved ones, even when distance separates us. Video calls, social media, and messaging apps allow us to maintain relationships with family and friends no matter where they are in the world. For those who may find it difficult to get out as often, online communities and interest groups can provide a sense of connection and community.

Virtual connections can complement face-to-face interactions, providing another way to stay in touch and share life's moments. Online book clubs, hobby groups, or even virtual exercise classes can be a great way to meet new people and expand your social network from the comfort of your home. While nothing replaces the warmth of in-person contact, digital tools can help bridge the gap when needed.

Building a Strong Social Foundation
Understanding the importance of social connections is the first step toward building a network that supports your well-being. By prioritizing meaningful relationships and making time for shared experiences, you can create a social life that enriches your daily routine and provides a sense of belonging. In the next section, we'll explore practical ways to strengthen bonds with family and friends, deepening the connections that matter most.

Strengthening Bonds with Family and Friends

Maintaining strong relationships with family and friends can bring a deep sense of fulfillment and support as we navigate life's changes. As we age, these relationships often take on new dynamics, whether it's adjusting to an empty nest, becoming a grandparent, or supporting aging parents. Strengthening these bonds requires effort, but the rewards sense of connection, shared experiences, and mutual support—are well worth it. Here are some practical ways to deepen your relationships with those closest to you.

1. Make Time for Regular Check-Ins
Life can be busy, even in retirement, but making time for regular check-ins with family and friends can help keep your relationships strong. Whether it's a weekly phone call with a friend, a standing lunch date with a sibling, or a monthly family dinner, these moments of connection provide an opportunity to catch up and share what's happening in each other's lives.

Consistency is key. Regular contact helps to maintain a sense of closeness, even when life gets hectic. It's also a way to show the people you care about that they are a priority in your life. If distance makes in-person visits difficult, technology can bridge the gap—video calls or group chats can make it easy to stay in touch, no matter where everyone is located.

2. Share Hobbies and Interests

Shared interests can be a wonderful way to bond with family and friends. Engaging in activities together creates a natural environment for conversation and laughter, building memories that strengthen your connection. If you and a friend enjoy reading, start a two-person book club and discuss your thoughts over coffee. If you share a love of gardening with a sibling, spend an afternoon tending to your plants together.

For those with children or grandchildren, finding activities that you can enjoy together—like baking, hiking, or crafting—can create special bonding moments. These shared experiences become treasured memories and help to foster a sense of togetherness across generations. It's not about the activity itself but the time spent enjoying each other's company.

3. Practice Active Listening

One of the most important aspects of deepening any relationship is the ability to listen actively. This means being fully present in conversations, giving your full attention, and showing empathy. Active listening involves not just hearing the words but also understanding the emotions behind them, which can strengthen the sense of connection between you and your loved ones.

When friends or family members share their thoughts and feelings, they resist the urge to offer advice right away. Sometimes, people just need to feel heard and validated. Respond with phrases like, "I understand how that might feel" or "Tell me more about that." This approach can deepen trust and create a safe space for open communication, helping to strengthen your relationships over time.

4. Show Appreciation and Gratitude
Expressing appreciation can go a long way in nurturing relationships. Taking the time to thank a friend for their support or letting a family member know how much you appreciate their company can strengthen bonds and foster a positive connection. It doesn't have to be elaborate—a heartfelt note, a small gift, or simply saying "thank you" can make a big difference.

Gratitude can also help shift the focus from what might be lacking in a relationship to the positive aspects that you value. For example, instead of focusing on a disagreement, take a moment to appreciate the qualities that drew you to your friend or family member in the first place. This perspective can help maintain a sense of warmth and appreciation, even during challenging times.

5. Create New Traditions
As life changes, old traditions may need to evolve, but that doesn't mean letting go of the joy of shared rituals. Creating new traditions with friends and family can help maintain a sense of connection and create something special to look forward to. This might be a monthly movie night with friends, an annual weekend getaway with siblings, or a new holiday ritual that includes everyone in the family.

For those with grandchildren, starting a special tradition— like a weekly storytelling session or a seasonal outing—can create cherished memories that last a lifetime. Traditions give a sense of continuity and belonging, reminding us of the people and experiences that matter most.

Building Stronger Bonds
Strengthening bonds with family and friends requires time, effort, and a willingness to be present. By making regular check-ins, sharing interests, practicing active listening, and showing appreciation, you can deepen the connections that provide a sense of support and joy in your life. In the next section, we'll explore how to expand your social circle by making new friends and building a sense of community, adding even more richness to your social life.

Making New Friends and Building Community

Making new friends and building a sense of community can enrich your life at any age. For women over 50, expanding social circles can offer new opportunities for connection, learning, and joy. Whether you're looking to meet new people in your neighborhood or through shared interests, cultivating new relationships can provide a sense of belonging and help combat feelings of isolation. Here are some practical ways to make new friends and create a vibrant community around you.

1. Join Local Clubs or Groups
One of the easiest ways to meet new people is by joining local clubs or interest groups. Many communities have book clubs, gardening societies, walking groups, and hobby clubs that welcome new members. These groups provide a natural way to meet others who share your interests, making it easier to strike up conversations and form connections.

If you're interested in learning a new skill or diving deeper into a hobby, consider taking a class at a community center or adult education program. Classes in cooking, painting, or even learning a new language can provide a structured environment where you can meet like-minded people. Plus, the shared experience of learning something new can be a great conversation starter.

2. Volunteer for a Cause You Care About

Volunteering is a wonderful way to give back to your community while also meeting new people. By working together on a shared cause, you can connect with others who have similar values and interests. Whether you're helping at a local animal shelter, serving meals at a food bank, or participating in community clean-up days, volunteering can create a sense of purpose and foster new friendships.

Many organizations actively seek volunteers of all ages, and they often provide training and support to help you get started. Volunteering can also introduce you to different age groups and backgrounds, providing a diverse social circle. It's a chance to build new connections while making a positive impact on the community around you.

3. Attend Community Events

Local events like farmers' markets, neighborhood festivals, art shows, or concerts in the park offer opportunities to meet new people in a relaxed setting. These events are often open to the public and attract a wide range of attendees, making it easy to strike up a conversation with a neighbor or fellow attendee.

If you're not sure where to start, look for community bulletin boards at your local library, grocery store, or community center, which often list upcoming events.

Attending these gatherings regularly can help you become familiar with a face, making it easier to start conversations and gradually build friendships. The key is to be open to new experiences and to say yes to invitations, even if they take you outside of your usual comfort zone.

4. Leverage Technology to Connect

In today's digital age, meeting new people doesn't have to be limited to in-person interactions. Online platforms like Meetup.com and local Facebook groups can help you find events and social gatherings that match your interests. Many online communities have formed around everything from hiking and cycling to book discussions and knitting circles.

Virtual meetups can also be a good way to get to know people before meeting in person. Joining an online group for a shared hobby or a virtual book club can help you connect with others, regardless of location. These digital connections can complement your in-person friendships, offering another way to stay socially active and engaged.

5. Be Open to Small Acts of Kindness

Sometimes, the simplest gestures can open the door to new friendships. Saying hello to a neighbor, complimenting someone's garden, or striking up a conversation while waiting in line can lead to unexpected connections. These small acts of kindness create opportunities to connect with others and can turn casual acquaintances into deeper friendships over time.

For those who find it difficult to approach new people, it can help to set small goals—like introducing yourself to one new person each week or inviting a neighbor over for tea. These small efforts can gradually build confidence and create a network of new connections. Remember, many people are looking for new friends just like you, and a little openness can go a long way.

Building a Community That Feels Like Home
Making new friends and building a sense of community can transform your experience of this stage of life. It's about being open to new experiences, finding people who share your interests, and trying to stay connected. In the next section, we'll explore how to navigate changes in relationships, whether it's adjusting to new dynamics with loved ones or letting go of relationships that no longer serve you.

Navigating Changes in Relationships

As we age, relationships often go through natural transitions. Changes in family dynamics, evolving friendships, and even shifts in romantic partnerships can create new challenges but also new opportunities for growth. Understanding how to navigate these changes with grace can help you maintain healthy connections and let go of those that no longer serve your well-being. Here are some strategies for managing the evolving nature of relationships during this stage of life.

1. Adjusting to Changes in Family Dynamics
Life events such as children leaving home, becoming grandparents, or caring for aging parents can significantly alter family relationships. The transition to an empty nest, for example, can bring about mixed emotions—pride in your children's independence, but also a sense of loss as your role shifts. Embracing this change as an opportunity to redefine your relationship with your adult children can

create a new dynamic that focuses on mutual respect and shared interests.

For those who become grandparents, this stage offers a chance to build a special bond with the next generation. However, it's important to find a balance between being involved and respecting the boundaries set by your children. Open communication can help clarify roles and expectations, ensuring that everyone feels comfortable and supported.

2. Navigating Friendship Changes

Friendships, like any relationship, can change over time as people's lives, interests, and priorities evolve. Sometimes, this means drifting apart from friends who once felt like family. While it can be painful to see a friendship fade, it's important to recognize that this is a natural part of life. Allow yourself to grieve the loss of a close friendship, but also be open to forming new connections that align with where you are now.

On the other hand, some friendships can deepen during this stage of life as shared experiences and understanding bring you closer together. Being open to change within friendships means finding new activities to enjoy together or adjusting how often you connect—can help maintain those relationships that remain meaningful. Flexibility and understanding are key to navigating the ebb and flow of friendships.

3. Rekindling Romance and Deepening Partnerships

Romantic relationships can also change as we age, whether it's adjusting to more time together after retirement or rediscovering your connection as you navigate new phases of life. For long-term partners, this stage can be an opportunity to deepen your bond, explore new interests together, and support each other's growth. It's a chance to redefine your relationship outside of previous roles, such as parents or caregivers, and focus on enjoying each other's company.

For those who find themselves single later in life, whether due to divorce or the loss of a partner, the idea of dating again can feel daunting. However, many people find that this stage of life offers a unique perspective on romance and the qualities they value in a partner. Approaching dating with an open heart and a sense of curiosity can lead to meaningful connections. Remember, it's never too late to find companionship or to redefine what love means to you.

4. Letting Go of Relationships That No Longer Serve You

Sometimes, the healthiest choice is to let go of relationships that have become toxic or no longer bring joy into your life. This can be especially true if a relationship is filled with negativity, constant conflict, or feelings of being drained rather than uplifted. Letting go can be difficult, especially if the relationship has been a part of your life for many years, but it's an important step in prioritizing your emotional well-being.

Setting boundaries is a crucial part of this process. It's okay to limit contact with people who make you feel stressed or unhappy. Focus on surrounding yourself with those who support your growth and bring positivity into your life. Sometimes, creating distance from certain relationships opens up space for new, healthier connections.

5. Seeking Support During Transitions

Navigating changes in relationships can bring up a lot of emotions—sadness, relief, uncertainty, and hope. It's important to remember that you don't have to go through these transitions alone. Seeking support from a trusted friend, counselor, or support group can provide a safe space to express your feelings and gain perspective. Talking through your experiences can help you process them more fully and find a way forward that feels right for you.

Change, though challenging, is often a gateway to personal growth. By embracing the natural evolution of relationships and focusing on those that bring you joy, you can create a social life that supports your well-being and happiness. In the next section, we'll explore the role of volunteering and giving back, and how contributing to your community can bring a sense of purpose and connection.

The Role of Volunteering and Giving Back

Volunteering and giving back to the community can provide a profound sense of purpose and fulfillment, especially as we age. Contributing to causes that matter to you not only benefits others but also enriches your own life, offering opportunities to connect, learn, and make a difference. For many women over 50, volunteering becomes a way to stay engaged with the world, build new relationships, and find meaning in everyday life. Here's how giving back can enhance your well-being and how to find the right opportunities for you.

1. Finding Purpose Through Service

Retirement or a shift in daily responsibilities can sometimes leave people feeling like they've lost a sense of purpose. Volunteering can fill this gap by providing meaningful activities that make a positive impact on the lives of others. Whether it's tutoring children, helping at a food pantry, or working with environmental groups, finding a cause that resonates with you can reignite a sense of purpose and accomplishment.

Many volunteers find that giving back is a way to channel their skills and experiences into something larger than themselves. For example, those with a background in teaching might enjoy mentoring students, while someone with a passion for gardening could help maintain community green spaces. The key is to find a role that aligns with your interests and values, making the experience both enjoyable and rewarding.

2. Building Connections Through Community Service
Volunteering is also an excellent way to meet new people and build connections. When you work alongside others who share your passion for a cause, it's easy to form friendships and create a sense of camaraderie. These connections can lead to deeper social ties and a feeling of being part of a larger community.

For many, the social aspect of volunteering becomes one of the most fulfilling parts of the experience. It provides a chance to meet people of all ages and backgrounds, broadening your perspective and bringing a sense of diversity to your social life. Whether you're helping organize a community event or working with a team to deliver meals to those in need, the shared effort can foster strong, lasting friendships.

3. Staying Active and Engaged
Volunteering often involves physical activity, which can help you stay active while doing good. Many volunteer opportunities, such as assisting at an animal shelter, participating in park clean-up efforts, or helping with local events, require movement and can provide a healthy way to stay active. This adds another layer of benefit, combining

physical activity with the emotional satisfaction of giving back.

Engaging in regular volunteer activities can also keep your mind sharp. The tasks involved—like planning events, problem-solving, or teaching—can provide a mental workout, helping to keep cognitive skills in shape. Volunteering can also stimulate creativity, offering a way to learn new skills or explore new interests.

4. Giving Back on Your Own Terms

Volunteering doesn't have to involve a large time commitment to make a difference. Even small acts of kindness can have a big impact. For example, knitting blankets for a local hospital, writing letters to isolated seniors, or donating time to read to children at a library are all meaningful ways to give back.

If mobility or time is a concern, consider virtual volunteering opportunities. Many organizations now offer roles that can be done from home, such as providing online tutoring, helping with social media for a non-profit, or making phone calls to check in on homebound seniors. These options allow you to contribute in a way that fits your lifestyle and comfort level.

5. Reflecting on the Impact of Your Efforts

One of the most rewarding aspects of volunteering is being able to see the positive impact of your efforts. Taking time to reflect on the difference you've made—whether it's the smile on a child's face, a cleaner park, or the gratitude of someone you've helped—can be a powerful reminder of the value of your time and energy. This sense of fulfillment can enhance your overall happiness and reinforce the benefits of staying connected to your community.

Many volunteers find that giving back helps them feel more connected to the world around them, fostering a sense of empathy and compassion. It's a way to give and receive at the same time, as the joy and appreciation you see in others often reflect back onto you.

Embracing the Joy of Service
Volunteering and giving back are more than just activities—they're ways to create meaning, build connections, and find joy in contributing to the well-being of others. By finding opportunities that align with your interests and values, you can make a positive impact on your community while enriching your own life. In the next chapter, we'll explore how to plan with confidence, focusing on financial wellness, retirement, and living with intention.

Chapter 8: Planning for the Future: Financial Wellness and Living with Intention

Building a Secure Financial Foundation

Financial wellness is a key part of living comfortably and confidently as we age. For many women over 50, managing finances can feel complex, especially when considering retirement, healthcare costs, and maintaining a lifestyle that supports well-being. Building a secure financial foundation doesn't have to be overwhelming—with careful planning and a focus on long-term goals, you can create stability and peace of mind for the years to come. Here's how to establish a solid financial base that supports your future.

1. Understanding Your Current Financial Picture
The first step to financial security is understanding where you currently stand. This involves taking stock of your income, expenses, savings, and any debt you might have. Reviewing your monthly budget can help you identify areas where you may be able to cut back, as well as opportunities to save more. Tracking expenses for a few months can reveal spending patterns and help you create a realistic budget that aligns with your priorities.

It's also important to review your assets, such as retirement accounts, investments, and real estate. This provides a clear picture of your financial resources and helps you determine whether adjustments are needed to meet your retirement goals. Working with a financial advisor can be beneficial, especially if you're uncertain about the best way to allocate your assets or want to ensure that your savings will last through retirement.

2. Prioritizing Savings and Emergency Funds

Even in retirement or semi-retirement, maintaining an emergency fund is essential. Life can be unpredictable, and having a cushion can help you manage unexpected expenses without dipping into long-term savings. Aim to keep three to six months' worth of living expenses in a separate, easily accessible account. This can cover unexpected costs like medical expenses, home repairs, or even unexpected travel needs.

Beyond an emergency fund, continuing to save for long-term goals is important, even if you're no longer working full-time. Consider allocating a portion of any part-time work, consulting income, or other earnings to savings or investments. The power of compounding interest means that even small contributions can grow over time, providing additional financial security as you age.

3. Managing Debt Wisely

Carrying debt into retirement can create additional financial stress, so it's important to address any existing debt before transitioning fully into retirement. Prioritize paying down high-interest debt, such as credit cards or personal loans, as these can quickly eat into your budget. If you have multiple debts, the "snowball method" (paying off the smallest debts first) or the "avalanche method" (tackling the highest interest debt first) can be effective strategies for reducing your financial burden.

If you have a mortgage, consider whether it makes sense to pay it off before retirement. For some, entering retirement without a mortgage can provide peace of mind, while others may benefit from keeping the mortgage for potential tax advantages. A financial advisor can help you weigh the pros and cons based on your individual situation.

4. Maximizing Social Security and Pensions

For many people, Social Security benefits and pensions are a significant part of retirement income. Understanding how to maximize these benefits can make a big difference in your overall financial picture. The age at which you start claiming Social Security can impact the amount you receive—waiting until full retirement age or even until age 70 can increase your monthly benefit significantly.

If you're eligible for a pension, review your options for taking payments. Some pensions offer a lump-sum payout, while others provide monthly payments for life. Consider factors such as your life expectancy, other sources of income, and your financial needs when deciding how to draw on these funds. Consulting with a retirement planner can help you make the best decision for your circumstances.

5. Investing for the Future

Investing can be a way to grow your savings, but it's important to adjust your investment strategy as you get closer to or enter retirement. A more conservative approach, with a focus on preserving capital, may be appropriate to reduce risk. This might mean shifting a portion of your investments from stocks to bonds or other stable assets that provide regular income.

Diversification remains key—by spreading investments across different asset classes, you can reduce the risk of any single investment impacting your financial security. For those who are not familiar with investing, working with a financial advisor can help you create a portfolio that aligns with your goals and risk tolerance.

Laying the Groundwork for Peace of Mind
Building a secure financial foundation takes time and
planning, but the effort pays off in the form of reduced
stress and greater confidence in your future. By
understanding your financial picture, prioritizing savings,
managing debt, and planning wisely for retirement income,
you can create a stable base that supports your lifestyle and
dreams. In the next section, we'll explore how to make the
most of your retirement years, turning this stage of life into
a time of growth, exploration, and fulfillment.

Retirement Planning: Making the Most of Your Time

Retirement is a time of significant change, offering the
freedom to explore new interests, deepen existing hobbies,
and enjoy more time with loved ones. While the transition
can bring excitement, it can also feel daunting without a
clear plan for how to fill your days. Approaching retirement
with a sense of purpose and intention can help ensure that
this chapter of life is both fulfilling and rewarding. Here's
how to plan for retirement in a way that makes the most of
your time and brings joy to your everyday routine.

1. Redefining What Retirement Means to You
The concept of retirement has changed significantly over
the years. For many, it's no longer just about stopping work
altogether, but about finding new ways to stay engaged and
active. Some people choose to pursue part-time work or
consulting opportunities, while others might explore
creative endeavors or volunteer roles. The key is to think
about what retirement means to you personally, whether
that's slowing down, staying active in your field, or
exploring a new passion.

Take some time to reflect on what you want your days to look like in retirement. What activities bring you joy? Are there projects you've always wanted to pursue but never had the time for? Defining your vision for retirement can help you create a plan that aligns with your goals and interests.

2. Exploring New Hobbies and Interests

Retirement offers the perfect opportunity to dive into hobbies you've always wanted to try or to rediscover interests that may have taken a backseat during your working years. Whether it's learning to paint, playing a musical instrument, or taking up gardening, having a variety of activities can keep your days rich with new experiences.

Consider joining local classes or community groups related to your interests, which can also be a great way to meet new people. If you enjoy staying active, trying out new physical activities like pickleball, yoga, or hiking can provide both a mental and physical boost. Exploring new hobbies isn't just about staying busy; it's about finding activities that make you feel excited to wake up each morning.

3. Planning for Travel and Adventure

For many, retirement is a time to explore the world, whether that means traveling to far-off destinations or discovering hidden gems closer to home. Planning for travel during retirement can be an exciting way to set goals and look forward to new experiences. Consider making a travel wish list, filled with places you've always wanted to visit or revisit.

Traveling doesn't have to mean long trips abroad; it can also be about exploring your own region or country.

Weekend getaways, road trips, and visiting national parks can provide a sense of adventure without the need for extensive planning. If budget is a concern, look for travel deals, consider house swapping, or explore volunteer tourism opportunities where you can give back while seeing new places.

4. Staying Connected with a Routine

While retirement offers freedom from a traditional work schedule, maintaining some form of routine can help you stay grounded and give structure to your days. A routine doesn't have to be rigid—it's more about creating a rhythm that supports your well-being and gives you a sense of purpose.

Your routine might include activities like morning walks, coffee with friends, time set aside for creative pursuits, or regular volunteer work. Even small rituals, like reading a chapter of a book each morning or taking time for afternoon tea, can create a comforting sense of structure. Having a routine can help prevent feelings of aimlessness and ensure that your time is spent on activities that enrich your life.

5. Finding Purpose in Giving Back

Many people find that retirement is an ideal time to give back to their communities in new ways. Volunteering can be a rewarding way to use your skills and experiences to make a difference, and it's also a great way to stay connected and engaged. Consider tutoring or mentoring young people, helping local nonprofits, or joining a community board.

Giving back doesn't have to be formal or time-consuming. It might mean offering to help neighbors, spending time with those who are isolated, or using your talents to support local causes. Many retirees find that volunteering adds a sense of purpose to their lives, allowing them to remain active and connected while contributing to the well-being of others.

Embracing a New Chapter
Retirement is not the end of your productive years—it's a new chapter filled with opportunities for growth, exploration, and joy. By defining what retirement means to you, staying active through hobbies, travel, and community engagement, and finding a routine that supports your lifestyle, you can create a retirement that is not just fulfilling, but truly meaningful. In the next section, we'll explore the benefits of downsizing and simplifying your life, making space for what truly matters.

Downsizing and Simplifying Your Life

As we move into new stages of life, simplifying our living spaces and letting go of excess can bring a sense of freedom and clarity. Downsizing doesn't have to mean giving up what you love, it's about creating a home that fits your current needs, making room for what truly matters. For many women over 50, downsizing can be a way to reduce stress, save money, and focus on experiences rather than possessions. Here's how to approach downsizing and simplifying your life in a way that feels positive and empowering.

1. Understanding the Benefits of Downsizing
Downsizing can offer a range of practical benefits, from lowering housing costs to making daily life more manageable. A smaller home often means lower utility bills, reduced maintenance, and less time spent cleaning

and upkeep. This can free up time and resources for the activities and experiences you value most, such as travel, hobbies, or spending time with loved ones.

Beyond the practical advantages, downsizing can also create a sense of mental and emotional clarity. Letting go of items that no longer serve a purpose can make your living space feel lighter and more peaceful. This process of simplifying can be particularly meaningful as you focus on what's most important in this stage of life, allowing you to live more intentionally.

2. Decluttering with a Purpose
The process of decluttering can feel overwhelming, especially if you've lived in the same home for many years. However, breaking the task into smaller, more manageable steps can make it easier. Start with one room or area at a time, sorting through items and deciding what to keep, donate, sell, or recycle. As you go through each item, ask yourself whether it still brings you joy or serves a purpose in your life.

For sentimental items that are difficult to part with, consider taking photos to preserve the memories without keeping the physical object. Passing down heirlooms to family members or friends can also be a way to share your legacy and keep those memories alive in a meaningful way. The goal is not to get rid of everything but to create a space that reflects who you are today.

3. Creating a Home That Suits Your Current Needs
As your lifestyle changes, your home should evolve to meet your new needs. This might mean moving to a smaller house or apartment, or simply rethinking the layout and function of your current space. For example, if you no

longer need a large dining room, consider turning that space into a hobby area, a reading nook, or a home office.

If mobility is a concern, downsizing can also be an opportunity to find a home that better supports accessibility, such as a one-story layout or a community with amenities designed for older adults. These changes can make daily life more comfortable and enjoyable, allowing you to focus on the things that bring you joy rather than worrying about home maintenance.

4. Embracing a Minimalist Mindset
Downsizing is not just about the physical process of moving or decluttering; it's also about embracing a minimalist mindset. This means focusing on what truly matters to you and letting go of the rest. Adopting a minimalist approach doesn't mean giving up everything you own, it's about being more intentional with what you keep and how you spend your time.

This mindset can extend beyond physical belongings to include your schedule and commitments. Simplifying your calendar by saying no to activities that no longer align with your priorities can create more time for the things that make you feel fulfilled. It's about making space—both physically and mentally—for the people, experiences, and activities that enrich your life.

5. Celebrating the Process of Letting Go
Downsizing and simplifying can be an emotional journey, especially when it involves letting go of items that hold sentimental value. It's normal to feel a sense of loss or nostalgia as you sort through memories. Allow yourself to feel those emotions without judgment, but also try to focus on the positive aspects of letting go—like the freedom that

comes with a less cluttered space or the joy of passing items on to others who can appreciate them.

Celebrate the progress you make along the way, no matter how small. Each item you let go of is a step toward creating a home that better reflects your current life. Take time to appreciate the newfound space and the opportunities it creates for new experiences and connections.

Living with Less, Loving It More
Downsizing and simplifying your life is about creating a living space that supports your happiness and well-being. By letting go of what no longer serves you, focusing on what you truly value, and embracing a minimalist mindset, you can create a home that feels peaceful, intentional, and ready for the next chapter. In the next section, we'll explore how to live with intention, setting goals for the future that align with your dreams and aspirations.

Living with Intention: Setting Goals for the Future

Living with intention means making choices that align with your values, dreams, and the life you envision for yourself. It's about being purposeful in how you spend your time, energy, and resources, creating a sense of fulfillment and meaning. As we age, living with intention becomes even more important, helping us to focus on what truly matters and let go of distractions. Here's how to set meaningful goals for the future and create a life that reflects your passions and aspirations.

1. Reflecting on Your Values and Priorities
The first step in living with intention is to understand your

core values—those things that are most important to you. Take some time to reflect on what brings you joy, what you're passionate about, and what you want to prioritize in this stage of life. Your values might include things like family, health, creativity, or giving back to the community.

Once you've identified your values, think about how you can align your daily life with them. For example, if health is a top priority, you might set goals around staying active or cooking nutritious meals. If building relationships is important to you, you might focus on spending more time with loved ones or joining social groups. These reflections can help you create goals that are deeply meaningful, guiding your decisions and actions in a way that feels authentic.

2. Setting SMART Goals

Setting goals that are specific, measurable, achievable, relevant, and time-bound (SMART) can help you turn your intentions into reality. Rather than setting vague goals like "get in shape" or "spend more time with family," SMART goals are clear and actionable. For example, "walk for 30 minutes, three times a week" or "have dinner with my grandchildren once a month" are goals that are easy to track and adjust as needed.

Breaking down larger goals into smaller steps can make them more manageable and increase the likelihood of success. Celebrate each milestone you reach, no matter how small, as these victories build momentum and keep you motivated. SMART goals can help you stay focused, making it easier to live intentionally and stay on track with the life you want to create.

3. Embracing a Growth Mindset

Living with intention is not about being perfect or

achieving every goal without setbacks. It's about adopting a growth mindset that you can continue to learn, grow, and improve at any age. A growth mindset helps you approach challenges with curiosity and resilience, seeing them as opportunities for self-discovery rather than as failures.

When working toward your goals, remind yourself that progress is more important than perfection. Be gentle with yourself if things don't go as planned and be willing to adjust your goals as your needs and desires change. This approach allows you to stay adaptable and open to new possibilities, making it easier to find joy in the journey itself.

4. Creating Daily Rituals That Reflect Your Intentions
Incorporating small, intentional rituals into your daily life can help you stay connected to your goals and values. These rituals don't have to be elaborate; they might include starting the day with a few moments of mindfulness, journaling your gratitude, or taking a daily walk to enjoy nature. These simple practices can serve as reminders of what's important to you, bringing a sense of purpose to even the most routine moments.

For many, rituals become a way to center themselves and create a sense of stability and peace. They provide a way to check in with yourself, ensuring that your actions are aligned with your intentions. By making these practices a regular part of your day, you can cultivate a lifestyle that feels intentional and deeply satisfying.

5. Looking Forward with Hope
Living with intention also means looking forward to the future with a sense of hope and optimism. It's about setting goals that excite you and dreaming about what's still possible. This might mean planning a trip, starting a new

creative project, or exploring a cause you care about. Allow yourself to think about the experiences and memories you still want to create.

Having something to look forward to can make each day feel more purposeful and give you the motivation to stay active and engaged. It's a reminder that this stage of life is full of potential, offering new opportunities for growth, learning, and joy. By keeping your eyes on the future while staying grounded in the present, you can create a life that feels rich with possibilities.

Designing a Life You Love
Living with intention means designing a life that reflects your deepest values and desires. By setting meaningful goals, embracing a growth mindset, and incorporating daily rituals that align with your vision, you can create a future that is both fulfilling and full of joy. In the next section, we'll explore legacy planning and how to leave a lasting impact on the people and communities you care about, ensuring that your values continue to shape the world around you.

Legacy Planning: Leaving a Lasting Impact

Legacy planning is about more than just finances; it's about creating a lasting impact on the people and causes that matter most to you. It's an opportunity to reflect on your values, share your wisdom, and leave a positive mark on the world. For many women over 50, thinking about the legacy they want to leave can provide a sense of purpose and help guide decisions about how to spend their time, resources, and energy. Here's how to approach legacy planning with intention, ensuring that your values continue to shape the lives of others.

1. Sharing Your Story and Wisdom

One of the most meaningful ways to leave a legacy is by sharing your life story and the lessons you've learned along the way. This might involve writing a memoir, recording your memories, or simply having conversations with loved ones about your experiences. These stories can become a cherished part of your family's history, offering insights into your values, challenges, and triumphs.

Consider creating a written or digital scrapbook that includes photos, letters, and stories that are important to you. This can be a beautiful way to pass down memories and keep your legacy alive for future generations. Even if you're not a writer, sharing your experiences verbally or through videos can be just as impactful, allowing your voice to reach those who may find comfort and guidance in your words.

2. Supporting Causes You Care About

Many people find meaning in supporting causes that align with their values and passions. Charitable giving, creating a scholarship, or donating to a cause you believe in are ways to make a difference that extends beyond your lifetime. If you have the means, setting up a charitable trust or foundation can provide ongoing support to the issues that matter to you, from education to environmental conservation.

Volunteering your time or skills can also be a part of your legacy. By mentoring young people, supporting local initiatives, or helping community organizations, you can make a direct impact on the lives of others. These acts of kindness and service can inspire those around you, creating a ripple effect that lasts long after you're gone.

3. Planning for Financial Legacy
While legacy planning often involves passing down assets, it's important to do so in a way that reflects your wishes and provides for the people you care about. This might mean creating a will, setting up trusts, or discussing your plans with an estate planner to ensure that your assets are distributed according to your wishes. Clear communication with your family about your plans can help prevent misunderstandings and ensure that your intentions are honored.

It's also important to consider how you want to approach end-of-life decisions. Having an advanced directive or living will can provide clarity about your healthcare preferences, ensuring that your wishes are respected even if you are unable to communicate them. Discussing these plans with your loved ones can provide peace of mind, knowing that your wishes will be honored.

4. Passing Down Traditions and Values
Beyond financial assets, passing down traditions, values, and skills can be an important part of your legacy. This might include teaching grandchildren how to cook a favorite family recipe, sharing stories about family traditions, or imparting the values that have guided you throughout your life. These intangible gifts can create a sense of continuity and help keep your memory alive in the hearts of those you love.

Consider writing letters to your children or grandchildren, offering advice, encouragement, and reflections on your hopes for their future. These letters can become treasured keepsakes, offering guidance and comfort during challenging times. By focusing on the values and traditions that matter most to you, you can leave a legacy that goes beyond material things, providing a source of inspiration for generations to come.

5. Living Your Legacy Every Day
Ultimately, the most powerful legacy you can leave is the one you create through your daily actions and interactions with others. Living with kindness, generosity, and integrity is a way of modeling the values you want to pass on, showing those around you what it means to live a life of purpose. Small gestures—like offering a listening ear, sharing a meal, or simply being present for others—can leave a lasting impression that shapes the lives of those you touch.

Reflect on how you want to be remembered and what qualities you hope to inspire in others. By living in alignment with those values each day, you can create a legacy that is already making a difference. Your actions today are a part of the legacy you leave behind, shaping how others remember you and the impact you've made on the world.

Creating a Lasting Impact
Legacy planning is a way to ensure that your values, stories, and passions continue to shape the world even after you're gone. By sharing your wisdom, supporting causes you care about, and focusing on the daily ways you can make a difference, you can create a legacy that reflects the life you've lived and the person you are. In the next chapter, we'll bring everything together, offering final reflections on embracing the art of aging gracefully and living a life filled with purpose, joy, and connection.

Chapter 9: Embracing the Journey: Final Reflections on Aging Gracefully

A Celebration of Wisdom and Experience

Aging is often seen through the lens of loss of youth, vitality, or the abilities we once took for granted. But another perspective reveals a different truth: aging is also a time to celebrate the wisdom and experience that come with a life fully lived. For women over 50, this stage of life offers the chance to reflect on the journey so far and to honor the knowledge, resilience, and growth that have been gained along the way. Embracing this celebration can transform how we view ourselves and our place in the world.

1. Honoring the Life You've Built
Looking back on the many roles you've played throughout your life—mother, partner, professional, friend, caregiver—it's clear that each chapter has shaped the person you are today. The experiences you've had, the challenges you've overcome, and the relationships you've built are all part of a rich tapestry that deserves to be celebrated. Taking time to reflect on the life you've created can bring a sense of pride and accomplishment.

This is a time to honor not only the achievements but also the struggles. Every setback and hardship have taught you something valuable about yourself and your capacity for resilience. Recognizing the strength it has taken to reach this point can be empowering, reminding you that you have the tools to continue facing whatever comes next.

2. Sharing Wisdom with the Next Generation

One of the gifts of growing older is the ability to share your wisdom with others, offering insights that only come with time and experience. Whether it's through mentoring younger colleagues, guiding your children or grandchildren, or simply being a source of support for friends, your perspective can be a valuable resource for those around you.

Sharing your wisdom doesn't mean having all the answers about offering understanding, empathy, and a willingness to listen. It's about letting others see that challenges are a normal part of life and that with patience and perseverance, they can be overcome. By being open about your own experiences, you can help others navigate their own paths with more confidence and clarity.

3. Embracing Your Unique Perspective

As we age, we often become more comfortable in our own skin, caring less about the opinions of others and more about what feels right for us. This sense of self-assurance is one of the greatest gifts of experience. It allows you to make decisions based on your own values and desires, rather than external pressures or expectations.

Embracing your unique perspective means being true to yourself in all aspects of life, from the choices you make to the way you spend your time. It's about letting go of the need for approval and focusing instead on what brings you joy and fulfillment. This freedom can be incredibly liberating, opening new possibilities for personal growth and happiness.

4. Finding Strength in Vulnerability

Celebrating wisdom also means embracing the strength that comes from vulnerability. As we grow older, we become more aware of our limitations and more accepting of the fact that we don't have to be perfect. This awareness can create space for deeper connections with others, as we become more willing to share our authentic selves without fear of judgment.

Being open about your fears, hopes, and uncertainties can strengthen relationships, allowing others to see the real you. It's a reminder that no one has to navigate life's challenges alone, and that the support we give and receive from others is a vital part of the human experience. Finding strength in vulnerability allows you to connect more deeply with those around you, creating bonds that are built on mutual trust and understanding.

5. Embracing the Beauty of Imperfection

Life is full of imperfections, but these imperfections are what make each person's story unique. Embracing the beauty of imperfection means accepting yourself as you are, flaws and all, and recognizing that growth is a lifelong process. It means appreciating the journey rather than focusing solely on the destination.

This perspective allows you to celebrate the wrinkles and gray hairs as signs of a life well-lived, rather than viewing them as losses. It's about seeing aging as a natural and beautiful part of the cycle of life, filled with opportunities to learn, grow, and love in new ways. By embracing the beauty of imperfection, you can find peace in the present and joy in the journey ahead.

A Life Worth Celebrating

Celebrating the wisdom and experience that come with age

is a way to honor the life you've built and the person you've become. It's a reminder that every stage of life has its own unique beauty and that there is value in the stories, lessons, and growth that each year brings. In the next section, we'll explore how to find joy in every stage of life, creating a mindset that allows you to appreciate the present while looking forward with hope and excitement.

Finding Joy in Every Stage of Life

Joy isn't reserved for a particular time in our lives, it's something we can cultivate at every stage, no matter what our age or circumstances. Finding joy as we age means focusing on what brings us happiness in the present, letting go of regrets about the past, and embracing a sense of curiosity and wonder about the future. For women over 50, this stage of life offers unique opportunities to rediscover joy in new ways, building a life that feels rich and fulfilling. Here's how to embrace joy in everyday moments and find delight in the process of aging.

1. Rediscovering Simple Pleasures
One of the gifts of aging is the ability to slow down and appreciate the simple pleasures of life. It's the quiet moments, like enjoying a cup of coffee on a sunny morning, listening to the laughter of grandchildren, or feeling the warmth of a loved one's embrace, that often bring the most joy. These small, everyday experiences become even more meaningful when we take the time to savor them fully.

Mindfulness can play a key role in rediscovering these simple pleasures. By being fully present in each moment, you can find beauty in the world around you, whether it's

in the changing colors of the seasons, the aroma of a
favorite meal, or the peacefulness of a quiet afternoon.
These moments of presence can be a source of deep
contentment, reminding you that joy is always within reach.

2. Staying Open to New Experiences

While it's natural to hold on to the activities and traditions
we've loved for years, staying open to new experiences can
bring unexpected joy and growth. This might mean trying a
new hobby, exploring a place you've never visited, or
simply saying yes to an opportunity that comes your way.
A willingness to embrace new experiences can keep life
feeling vibrant and exciting, no matter your age.

Being open to new things doesn't have to be about grand
adventures—it can be as simple as trying a new recipe,
learning to play an instrument, or taking a class at a local
community center. These experiences provide a sense of
novelty and challenge that can reignite your curiosity and
sense of wonder. They also offer opportunities to meet new
people and make new connections, adding richness to your
social life.

3. Cultivating Gratitude for the Present

Gratitude is a powerful tool for finding joy, helping to shift
your focus from what's missing in life to what's already
abundant. By making a habit of expressing gratitude, you
can train your mind to notice the positive aspects of each
day, even during difficult times. This practice doesn't just
lift your spirits in the moment—it can also build a more
positive outlook over time.

Consider keeping a gratitude journal, where you write
down a few things you're thankful for each day. These
entries don't have to be grand or life-changing—they might
include a kind word from a friend, a beautiful sunset, or the

feeling of accomplishment after a walk. Looking back on these entries can remind you of the many moments of joy that have woven through your life, creating a sense of appreciation for the present.

4. Finding Joy in Connection

Joy is often found in connection with others—whether it's through deep conversations, shared laughter, or simply spending time together. Nurturing relationships with friends, family, and community can provide a sense of belonging and emotional support, which is especially important as we age. Making time for regular social activities, from coffee dates to group outings, can keep you feeling engaged and connected.

For those who may live alone or feel isolated, seeking out new social opportunities can open the door to new friendships and experiences. Joining a club, taking part in local events, or even volunteering can be ways to build connections that add joy and meaning to your days. It's a reminder that joy is not only something we find within ourselves but also something that grows when shared with others.

5. Embracing a Sense of Playfulness

A sense of playfulness doesn't have to fade with age—in fact, it can become an even more cherished part of life as we grow older. Embracing playfulness means allowing yourself to be silly, to laugh without reserve, and to find delight in the unexpected. It's about reconnecting with the childlike wonder that allows you to see the world with fresh eyes.

Playfulness might mean dancing to your favorite songs in the living room, exploring a new art form, or spending time with children and letting their enthusiasm rub off on you.

It's about finding moments of lightness and fun in your everyday life, and not taking yourself too seriously. This sense of joy can add a youthful energy to your days, reminding you that it's never too late to enjoy life's simple pleasures.

Finding Joy in the Journey
Finding joy in every stage of life is about embracing the present, staying open to new experiences, and celebrating the connections that make life rich. By focusing on what brings happiness into your life today, you can create a sense of fulfillment that carries you forward with a joyful heart. In the next section, we'll explore how to build a legacy of love and connection, ensuring that the joy you create extends far beyond yourself.

Building a Legacy of Love and Connection

Creating a legacy isn't just about material wealth or achievements, it's about the love, wisdom, and kindness you share with others throughout your life. For women over 50, building a legacy of love and connection means focusing on the relationships that matter most, nurturing bonds with family and friends, and finding ways to make a positive impact on those around you. This kind of legacy is one that can be felt in the hearts of those you touch, offering comfort, guidance, and inspiration for years to come. Here's how to build a legacy that celebrates love and connection.

1. Prioritizing Relationships with Loved Ones
One of the most powerful aspects of your legacy is the way you nurture your relationships with the people closest to you. This might mean making time for regular family

gatherings, organizing outings with friends, or simply
calling or visiting those who mean the most to you. These
small acts of connection create lasting memories and
remind your loved ones that they are a priority in your life.

For those with children or grandchildren, creating special
traditions—like weekly dinners, holiday celebrations, or
shared hobbies—can strengthen bonds and create a sense of
continuity across generations. These moments become
cherished rituals that family members will remember and
carry forward, keeping your spirit alive in their own lives.

2. Sharing Stories and Life Lessons
The stories you share and the lessons you've learned over a
lifetime can be a valuable part of your legacy. Whether it's
tales from your childhood, insights from your career, or
reflections on how you've overcome challenges, these
stories can offer wisdom and guidance to those who come
after you. Sharing these lessons can help others navigate
their own journeys with a little more confidence and clarity.

Consider writing down some of your stories or recording
them in audio or video format. This can be a way for your
family to revisit your voice and memories, even after
you're gone. You might also write letters to loved ones,
offering words of encouragement, advice, and love that
they can keep as a source of comfort and inspiration. These
personal messages can become treasured keepsakes, a way
for your voice to continue guiding those you care about.

3. Leading by Example in Kindness and Compassion
A legacy of love is built through everyday acts of kindness
and compassion. By showing empathy to others, offering a
helping hand, and treating people with respect, you set an
example that inspires those around you. This approach to
life can become a model for your children, grandchildren,

and friends, showing them the power of treating others with care and understanding.

It's not about grand gestures, it's about the small, consistent acts of kindness that leave a lasting impression. Offering to help a neighbor, listening without judgment, or simply smiling at a stranger can all make a difference. These actions create a ripple effect, encouraging others to spread kindness in their own lives and helping to create a more compassionate world.

4. Volunteering and Community Involvement

Another way to build a legacy of connection is through service to your community. Volunteering your time, sharing your expertise, or mentoring young people can create a sense of purpose while making a positive impact on those around you. Community involvement allows you to leave a tangible mark on the places you care about, whether it's through supporting a local organization, helping to organize events, or simply being a steady presence in your neighborhood.

Community service is a way to pass on your values to future generations, showing that a fulfilling life includes giving back to others. It's a reminder that we are all part of something larger than ourselves, and that the love and energy we invest in our communities can continue to flourish long after we're gone.

5. Leaving a Legacy of Love Through Presence

Ultimately, the greatest legacy you can leave is your presence in the lives of those you love. It's about showing up for the important moments, being there to support friends and family during challenges, and celebrating their successes. It's the way you make people feel heard, valued, and cherished that stays with them long after the words have faded.

Being fully present with others means giving them your time and attention, putting aside distractions, and listening with an open heart. These moments of presence create deep connections that leave a lasting impact. They remind those you care about that they are not alone, that they are seen and appreciated. This kind of love is a gift that continues to shape lives, creating a legacy that is felt, not just remembered.

A Legacy That Lives On
Building a legacy of love and connection is about focusing on the relationships and actions that bring meaning to your life. By sharing your stories, leading with kindness, and being present for those you love, you can create a legacy that leaves a lasting impression on the hearts of others. In the next section, we'll explore how to look ahead with hope and positivity, embracing the future with a mindset that welcomes new possibilities.

Looking Ahead with Hope and Positivity

Aging gracefully means embracing each new stage of life with hope and positivity, focusing on the opportunities that lie ahead rather than dwelling on what has passed. This mindset can help transform how you experience the future, allowing you to face challenges with resilience and appreciate the joys that each day brings. For women over 50, looking ahead with hope is about remaining open to new possibilities, finding ways to stay engaged, and nurturing a sense of optimism. Here's how to cultivate a hopeful and positive outlook as you move forward.

1. Focusing on Possibilities, Not Limitations

It's natural to notice the changes that come with aging, whether they're physical, emotional, or social. But instead of focusing on what might be more difficult, try to shift your perspective to what's still possible. This might mean exploring new hobbies, learning a skill you've always been curious about, or simply allowing yourself to dream about what you'd like to accomplish in the years to come.

A mindset focused on possibilities allows you to approach each day with curiosity and a sense of adventure. It's a reminder that growth doesn't stop at any age, and that there's always something new to discover or experience. By embracing the idea that the future holds potential for joy and fulfillment, you can keep a sense of excitement and wonder alive.

2. Practicing Self-Compassion

Looking ahead with hope also means being kind to yourself, especially on difficult days. Self-compassion involves recognizing that aging comes with challenges, and that it's okay to have moments of doubt or sadness. By treating yourself with the same empathy you would offer a friend, you can navigate these feelings without letting them overshadow your optimism.

Self-compassion can be as simple as giving yourself permission to rest when you need it, celebrating small victories, or acknowledging the effort you've put into caring for yourself and others. It's about focusing on progress rather than perfection and being patient with yourself as you adapt to changes. This approach creates a sense of inner peace that supports a more hopeful outlook on life.

3. Staying Inspired by Role Models

Finding inspiration in others who are aging gracefully can be a powerful way to cultivate hope. Look for role models who embody the values and mindset you aspire to—whether they are authors, community leaders, friends, or family members. Seeing how others have found meaning and joy in their later years can remind you that this stage of life is full of potential.

Books, interviews, and articles featuring stories of people who have thrived in their later years can provide motivation and ideas for your own journey. Learning about others' experiences can open your mind to new possibilities and help you see aging as a time of opportunity rather than decline.

4. Embracing a Growth Mindset

A growth mindset—the belief that you can continue to learn and grow throughout your life—can help you face the future with optimism. This mindset encourages you to see challenges as opportunities for growth, and to believe that new skills and abilities can be developed at any age. It's about embracing change and staying open to new ways of thinking.

For example, if you encounter a physical limitation that makes an activity more difficult, a growth mindset might encourage you to try a modified version or explore an entirely new activity. It's not about ignoring the realities of aging, but about focusing on what you can do, rather than what you can't. This shift in perspective can create a sense of empowerment, helping you approach the future with confidence.

5. Finding Joy in the Present Moment

Hope and positivity are grounded in the ability to find joy

in the present moment. By focusing on what's good in your life right now, you can cultivate a sense of contentment that supports a positive outlook. This might involve practicing gratitude, spending time with loved ones, or engaging in activities that bring you a sense of peace and satisfaction.

Mindfulness practices, such as meditation or simply taking time to appreciate nature, can help you stay grounded in the present. These practices remind you that the future is built on the moments you live each day, and that by finding joy in those moments, you can create a life that feels meaningful and fulfilling.

Embracing a Bright Tomorrow
Looking ahead with hope and positivity means embracing the unknown with a sense of curiosity and trust. By focusing on possibilities, practicing self-compassion, and staying open to new experiences, you can create a future that is rich with meaning and joy. In the final section, we'll explore what it truly means to embrace the art of aging gracefully, bringing together the themes of love, connection, and self-care into a vision for a vibrant and fulfilling life.

Embracing the Art of Aging Gracefully

Aging gracefully isn't about trying to turn back the clock or denying the changes that come with time. Instead, it's about finding peace with the process, embracing each new stage of life, and celebrating the person you've become. It means focusing on the beauty of your unique journey and recognizing that every line, every story, and every lesson learned is a testament to a life lived with heart and soul. For women over 50, embracing the art of aging gracefully can be a transformative experience, allowing you to approach the future with a sense of openness, gratitude, and self-love.

1. Accepting Yourself as You Are

The first step to aging gracefully is accepting yourself as you are—embracing the changes in your body, your appearance, and your abilities with compassion and understanding. This acceptance doesn't mean giving up on caring for yourself; rather, it means doing so from a place of love rather than pressure. It's about celebrating your body for all it has done for you and continues to do, rather than focusing on what it no longer does in the same way.

When you let go of the need to fit into a certain image or meet external expectations, you can begin to see yourself through a kinder, more forgiving lens. Acceptance allows you to focus on what truly makes you feel good, whether that's a nourishing skincare routine, a comfortable wardrobe that makes you feel beautiful, or daily movement that keeps you feeling strong.

2. Finding Meaning in Connection

Aging gracefully also involves staying connected to the people and communities that bring meaning to your life. Relationships with family, friends, and neighbors can provide a sense of belonging and support, enriching your daily experience. As you focus on nurturing these connections, you'll find that the love and joy shared with others become some of the most precious gifts of this stage of life.

Whether it's through mentoring younger generations, volunteering in your community, or simply spending time with friends, these connections help keep your spirit alive. They remind you that you are part of a larger story and that the impact of your life continues to ripple outward through the people you touch.

3. Living in Harmony with Change

Change is a constant, but learning to live in harmony with it can make the process of aging feel more natural and less intimidating. This means embracing the ebb and flow of life, accepting that there will be moments of loss and sadness, but also times of great joy and discovery. Rather than resisting these changes, try to find a rhythm that allows you to flow with them, adapting as needed while staying true to yourself.

Living in harmony with change also means giving yourself permission to let go of what no longer serves you. This might include outdated goals, old habits, or even relationships that no longer bring positivity into your life. By releasing these, you create space for new experiences and connections, allowing your life to evolve in ways that feel true to who you are now.

4. Cultivating a Sense of Gratitude and Joy

Gratitude and joy are the cornerstones of aging gracefully. They allow you to focus on the abundance in your life, rather than what might be lacking. Gratitude turns ordinary moments into celebrations, and joy helps you find delight in the little things, from a walk in the park to a quiet moment with a loved one.

A daily gratitude practice—whether it's writing down what you're thankful for or simply taking a moment to appreciate the beauty around you—can transform how you experience each day. It's a reminder that even in the midst of challenges, there is always something to be grateful for. This perspective can help you approach life with an open heart, making each day feel like a gift.

5. Embracing the Journey with Courage and Grace
Aging gracefully is ultimately about approaching each day with courage and grace. It's about being brave enough to face the unknown, to embrace vulnerability, and to continue growing. It means recognizing your own strength and using it to navigate life's changes with a sense of calm and dignity.

Grace comes from accepting that life's beauty is often found in its imperfections, and courage comes from knowing that you have the power to create a meaningful and fulfilling life, no matter your age. By embracing this mindset, you can find peace with the past, joy in the present, and hope for the future.

A Life of Beauty and Wisdom
Embracing the art of aging gracefully is a journey that invites you to live with authenticity, kindness, and a deep appreciation for the life you've lived. It's about finding meaning in every stage, celebrating your unique path, and continuing to look forward with hope and excitement. By choosing to age with grace, you honor not only the person you have been but the person you are becoming, creating a life that is truly beautiful in every sense.

Thank You!

Thank you so much for reading *Grace in Every Season: A Guide to Thriving After 50*. I hope this book has inspired you to embrace each stage of life with a renewed sense of joy, confidence, and self-love. It's been a privilege to share this journey with you, and I truly hope the insights and stories on these pages have been a source of comfort and inspiration.

If *Grace in Every Season* has resonated with you, I would be incredibly grateful if you could take a few moments to leave a review on Amazon. Your feedback helps other readers discover the book and allows me to continue sharing stories and insights with the community. Simply visit Amazon and share your thoughts—I'd love to hear from you!

Thank you again for being a part of this journey. May you continue to thrive and find grace in every season of your life.

With gratitude,
Thomas Buchheister

www.ingramcontent.com/pod-product-compliance
Lightning Source LLC
Chambersburg PA
CBHW052018150726

47999CB00004B/1717